THE DEEP BLUE SLEEP

"*The Deep Blue Sleep* is not just a book—it's a transformative journey towards better sleep, enhanced vitality, and renewed quality of life. Whether you're struggling with insomnia, sleep apnea, or simply seeking to optimize your sleep, this book is an indispensable companion. Dr. Corca's clear and empathetic voice navigates readers through the multifaceted landscape of sleep issues, providing invaluable insights, personalized strategies, and making complex concepts accessible and actionable."

—**Dr. Izabella Wentz**, PharmD, FASCP, *New York Times* Bestselling Author *Hashimoto's Protocol*

"*The Deep Blue Sleep* book offers a unique and valuable perspective on how to heal insomnia naturally. Now more than ever, our patients need help decreasing stress and the many other things interrupting a restorative sleep pattern. Dr. Corca's knowledge, along with her companionate and individualized approach, covers not only the basics but also the complex challenges that affect men and women. This book is a must-read on how to hack the foundation component of wellness, a great night's sleep!"

—**Dr. Jill Carnahan**, MD, Functional Medicine Practitioner, Teacher, Bestselling Author of *Unexpected*

"Poor sleep accelerates disease. Good sleep accelerates healing. *The Deep Blue Sleep* book offers a holistic view into the world of sleep and how to improve sleep naturally. A terrific guide for anyone with sleep issues looking for a holistic approach to having better sleep."

—**Dr. Terry Wahls**, MD, IFMCP, Bestselling Author of *The Wahls Protocol—A Radical New Way to Treat All Chronic Autoimmune Conditions Using Paleo Principles*

"Dr. Damiana Corca's book, *The Deep Blue Sleep*, represents a fresh approach in the realm of sleep health and wellness. With a deep understanding of the interconnectedness of the body's systems and traditional medicine, she offers readers a clear and actionable roadmap to achieving the restorative sleep they deserve. She not only educates readers on the importance of good sleep but also empowers them to take control of their sleep health. Dr. Corca's years of clinical experience shine through as she provides practical solutions tailored to each insomniac type. *The Deep Blue Sleep* is hope for those who have struggled with sleepless nights. It is a must-read for anyone seeking solutions for better sleep."

—**Dr. Alan Christianson**, NMD, *New York Times* Bestselling Author of *The Thyroid Reset Diet*

"It is well established today that sleep is vital to health. Although *The Deep Blue Sleep* is meant to address the layperson, I find that it contains a wealth of information for the professional as well. Damiana Corca's text helps the layperson easily identify their insomnia pattern with practical advice and strategies for dealing with their particular issues. A book that I recommend both to patients and colleagues."

—**Dr. Hamid Montakab**, MD, Acupuncturist, Internationally Recognized Teacher, Author of *Acupuncture for Insomnia*

"Sleep is the golden thread that supports our mental and physical well-being. *The Deep Blue Sleep* provides a natural solution with functional guidance that is needed in our society, with sleep issues becoming a growing concern and affecting cognition, healing, mood, and our ability to access happiness and peace. Dr. Corca provides knowledgeable and compassionate insight and expert advice, inviting replenishing nights of sleep. This will be a valuable addition to your personal library and any health practitioner's office now and in the future."

—**Melissa Wolak**, MS, CCC-SLP, CTP, Speaker, Therapeutic Coach and Speech-Language-Cognitive Therapist

"*The Deep Blue Sleep* is a groundbreaking book on healing sleep from a truly holistic perspective. The unique five insomnia types model easily guides you toward the underlying cause of why you can't sleep well and what to do to sleep soundly night after night."

—**Dr. Jolene Brigthen**, NMD, Leader in Women's Health, Speaker, Bestseller Author of *Beyond the Pill*

"Dr. Damiana Corca has been a lifesaver for many of my patients over the years. She has a unique knowledge base and skill set, which she has chosen to share with us in *The Deep Blue Sleep* book. Let this book be the beginning of your journey to the land of better sleep. I also highly recommend working with her in person to experience her healing presence and acupuncture skills—she works magic!"

—**Dr. Jennifer Johnson**, MD, Family Physician, Boulder, Colorado

"Dr. Damiana Corca invites us to do a deep dive within ourselves. Her exciting new book, *The Deep Blue Sleep*, takes us on a multidisciplinary journey into understanding our bodies and our minds. With warmth, compassion, and expertise, Damiana takes our hand and walks with us on our journey to better understand ourselves. Along the way, she teaches us about sleep, stress, inflammation, infections, wellness, and how they all come together. The result is better sleep, better health, better living. I recommend my patients work with Damiana, and I recommend they also read her book."

—**Dr. Kevin Lutz**, MD, FACP, Founder of Concierge Medical Care in Denver, Colorado, Assistant Clinical Professor at the University of Colorado School of Medicine and Kansas City University

THE DEEP BLUE SLEEP

A ROADMAP TO FALL ASLEEP AND STAY ASLEEP NATURALLY

DR. DAMIANA CORCA

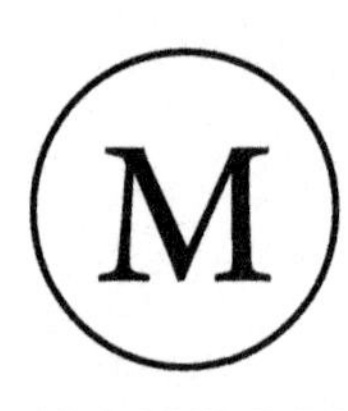

MANUSCRIPTS
PRESS

COVER ART BY LAURA BEE

THE DEEP BLUE SLEEP
A Roadmap to Fall Asleep and Stay Asleep Naturally

ISBN 979-8-88926-554-2 *Paperback*
979-8-88926-555-9 *Ebook*

To all the people who are tired of not being able to sleep well and not understanding why they can't sleep, I hope this book will bring you the clarity and healing that you have been waiting for.

CONTENTS

PREFACE

The longest years of my life were around the time I attended high school. As a teenager, I felt like I was forgotten by God, and it was by some sad mistake that I ended up growing up on a farm in the middle of nowhere in Transylvania (Romania). Part of it was because there was lots of work on the farm. During the school year, I was gone to school at least part of the day, but the three-month summer vacation was the most challenging, working the land and tending to the animals from 6 a.m. to 10 p.m. The light at the end of the tunnel was graduating high school and going to college.

The only escape from my life was nighttime. This was my time to dream and fantasize. I would let the radio play all night to mostly foreign songs I barely understood the words to. I counted on the music to wake me up intermittently so I could lengthen this time that was all mine. If I slept through the night, I was sorely disappointed in the morning. I had infinite satisfaction in those short moments of awareness, of stealing time that was forbidden.

I never realized back then that I was causing myself what I now know is insomnia. But what I have learned from this is that sleeping well doesn't look the same for everyone, and getting better doesn't look the same either. This type of thinking can create a better terrain to facilitate the healing process. Mindset is incredibly important since it affects the way we react and the way our body responds.

Suffering from insomnia is hard. Day in and day out, I speak with patients who say they feel frustrated and angry at times, and at other times break down crying out of hopelessness and desperation. It can be a lonely experience lying in bed during the darkest part of the night, all alone, filled with anxiety and dread. Sleeping well one night, only to sleep terribly the next can heighten anxiety and exacerbate insomnia. Regardless, they continue to work on improving their health with the hope that sleep will finally come.

This book will give you that understanding so you feel empowered and can react less if and when you have a less-than-ideal night of sleep. What I've learned over the past fourteen years is that you can only treat a problem once you understand what, exactly, is causing it. This book attempts, to the best of my ability, to present what I see happening in people who struggle with sleep.

The resources to heal are out there, but if you don't know what to treat, working on healing insomnia can feel hopeless.

A good night of sleep doesn't start when you climb into bed, nor can you rely on a nightly wind-down routine to solve all your sleep problems. Proper rest requires establishing a good sleep environment and attaining a healthy functioning nervous system, which begins the moment we wake up.

This book is for people who have trouble sleeping on their own, are tired of being tired, and are interested in finding a solution to their sleep struggles within natural medicine. Finding the root cause of your insomnia will not only help you heal your sleep but will also help improve your overall health. It will help you feel more empowered to understand what happens in your body when you experience sleep troubles.

My deepest hope is that this book offers what the color blue in the title suggests—a feeling of calmness and relaxation calling us to our natural state. May the serene blue sky and the calm blue sea instill a sense of peace, safety, and tranquility to give you the deepest and most restful sleep, night after night.

INTRODUCTION

What is good sleep?

Before going into what can go wrong with sleep, it is helpful to understand what good sleep is. Good sleep means different things to different people. But I think we can all agree on these three primary parameters:

Sleep initiation: It's easy to fall asleep when you go to bed.

Sleep continuation: You sleep through the night or wake up once and go back to sleep easily.

Sleep quality: You wake up feeling refreshed and have good energy throughout the day.

All else from here on is a variation of these three parameters. Good sleep is when you sleep seven and a half to nine hours per night. We tend to sleep in ninety-minute cycles, so that would give us five to six cycles. The people who sleep six hours and feel well are rare. Check out the online bonus genetics chapter. As you lie in bed, it takes you no longer than thirty minutes to fall asleep—ideally ten to twenty—and not faster than ten minutes. If it takes too long to fall asleep, you have onset insomnia; if it takes too little time, you are likely sleep deprived.

It's a healthy sign when you feel sleepy and groggy as you approach the time you go to bed rather than feeling tired but wired. Then when you wake up in the morning, you feel relaxed and peaceful rather than stressed and wired, or depressed.

You should wake up feeling energized and refreshed, like you had a nice, long, deep sleep. If you wake up at night, it's only briefly, and you are able to go back to sleep. In some situations, some people may be up for an hour or so. If you don't have anxiety or worry, you actually enjoy it, and you meet all the other criteria I mention here, then by all means, you are likely doing just fine and don't need to change anything.

Waking up once to urinate can be expected, even twice for older individuals. However, anything above that needs to be looked into, as it is likely affecting the quality of your sleep. You may need to decrease your water intake in the evening, or your urinary function requires support.

Dreaming is good and normal; however, if it leaves you tired or is too vivid and disturbing, that should be addressed as the dreams are likely affecting your sleep and functioning the next day.

As a healthy sleeper, you should sleep through the night without feeling hungry or thirsty. If you feel hungry, you might need to make dietary changes or may possibly have a blood sugar imbalance. Feeling thirsty in the middle of the night can be normal for some people, or it may mean you need to hydrate better during the day or that you need to look into the healing of your hormones. Women who have hot flashes and night sweats as well as older individuals tend to feel thirsty at night, usually not relieved by drinking more water during the day.

Your breathing should be regular, without gasping for air, and you shouldn't have interrupted breathing throughout the night, directly noticed by you or your bed partner.

It is normal to have a slight decrease in energy in the early afternoon, though you should have enough energy to easily keep going. Typically, your energy picks up again later in the afternoon.

More critical than exactly how many hours you sleep and how, exactly, your night looks is how you feel when you wake up and during the day. If you feel well as you wake up, remain energized and focused throughout the day, and start feeling a significant drop in energy only a couple of hours before your bedtime, you are most likely getting enough good sleep.

I have built a resource page on my website for information I wanted to share with you that was too lengthy to share in this book. You can find this page at damianacorca.com/resources.

PART I

THE FIVE INSOMNIAC TYPES

Part I introduces you to the five insomniac types framework. Understanding which type you are will help you identify which chapters in the book may be more pertinent to your sleep healing journey.

CHAPTER ONE

IDENTIFYING YOUR TYPE

Knowing the main types of insomnia that people commonly suffer from will set the stage for explaining how to heal.

Unfortunately, the more simplistic way of categorizing insomnia, *onset insomnia* and *maintenance insomnia,* falls short regarding the healing process.

In my clinical practice, I have concluded that there is much more to insomnia than "I can't fall asleep" or "I can't stay asleep."

The work of Hamid Montakab, MD, opened my mind to a new way of looking at the many types of insomnia from the Chinese Medicine perspective. His book *Acupuncture for Insomnia: Sleep and Dreams in Chinese Medicine* is the foundation of my Chinese medicine clinical practice. Chinese Medicine combines acupuncture, herbs, and nutrition to help heal a patient holistically.

After hearing so many stories of how insomnia is expressed in each person, I can clearly see patterns that have common roots. Insomnia is not random. For the people living with insomnia who have been at it for decades, nothing is more disheartening than being told you have maintenance insomnia, and here, try some sleep hygiene and perhaps an herb or a medication.

At the very least, we want someone to understand the complexity of our sleep and validate our struggle. We tend to blame ourselves when we hit a wall without a real explanation for our insomnia. *Something must be wrong with me, with my body.* That is a hard place to be in, especially because our struggle happens at night when we are all alone.

The five types of insomnia presented in the following pages have their own characteristics but are also deeply interconnected. Differentiating between them helps us find a path to healing more clearly. It helps me, as the practitioner, to identify the root cause so we can confidently focus on healing insomnia and avoid getting sidetracked when the progress is slower than we would like.

Understanding which type of insomnia you suffer from is more likely to help us find out why insomnia develops in the first place, and once you heal, to understand how to prevent relapses.

The five types are the following: **the anxious type, the overthinking type, the overtaxed type, the depleted type, and the overburdened type.**

The first three are the most common types of insomnia I see in the clinic. Symptoms associated with these three types are most commonly present in patients suffering from sleep struggles. Some people have a combination of two types but experience one type more often. Also, the type of insomnia you experience may change throughout the years.

Identifying your type

Understanding the five types of insomnia can help you figure out how to heal. Some people may experience the same type of insomnia when stress is more intense than their nervous system can handle, but otherwise, they sleep well.

We may suffer from one type in our twenties and another in our forties. These are not meant as a permanent label you want to be attached to but rather *to provide a framework to guide healing.*

If you have had mild insomnia on and off, understanding these types and their root cause will help you avoid developing chronic insomnia by addressing it now before it becomes part of your life. On the other hand, if you have chronic insomnia, this will help you identify which category you fit in so the Healing section will be more approachable.

Suppose you have an apparent inclination toward being a night owl or an early bird, which is likely due to genetic tendencies. There is a fine line between differentiating what is a genetic tendency, what is just a developed habit, like staying up late consistently, and what is an actual pathology. For example, women with PCOS—polycystic ovarian syndrome—often think they are night owls, but when they heal the root cause of PCOS, their clock shifts, and they can fall sleep earlier.

As you read all five types, notice the various other parts of the body that may be affected. You will learn that insomnia is not typically a disease that happens on its own but rather is a combination of other symptoms that may seem unrelated in your mind.

As we look at the whole person, we see how the body shifts from a healthy to a diseased state. Every time we feel unwell, it's simply a warning signal that something is off, and the body can no longer compensate. Ideally, we get to know our body so well that we notice the little signs when something is heading in an unhealthy direction. My aim with this book is to describe many of these signs so you can observe them in your daily life before your entire body screams for help.

Life can feel so busy, filled with external distractions. When we experience a minor headache here and there, a mild tummy cramp when eating, something a bit off with the hormones, an occasional bad night of sleep, and so on, we tend to ignore these and keep going. We don't want to be hypochondriacs. But if we don't listen now, we will listen later. I often wish my patients would come in for help when their problem with sleep was about half the intensity they experienced when they came to see me. They would have suffered less, and the healing progress would have been faster.

Read all five types before determining which type your insomnia falls into. Then in the healing chapters, various symptoms associated with the main systems affected will help you better understand your type.

CHAPTER TWO

THE ANXIOUS TYPE

"If I do things just right—maybe—I will fall asleep."

That's what the anxious type will say when they have trouble initiating sleep. Anxiety associated with insomnia is found, to a certain degree, in all types of insomniacs. But it is undoubtedly more common in some people. Once you feel anxious, your ability to fall asleep worsens, which in turn exacerbates the anxiety. And so the negative loop keeps going.

Anna was a forty-two-year-old new mom. Her baby girl was almost two years old when she came into my office. Anna's insomnia started when her baby was born. Her newborn had frequent acid reflux, and she would wake up every half an hour or so each night for the first six months of her life.

Fortunately, between six and nine months old, her baby started sleeping better and for longer periods of time. Unfortunately, Anna realized that she now had insomnia. She tried medications and worked with a holistic practitioner, which helped her insomnia move from absolutely terrible to at least sort of manageable.

I still remember when she walked into my office. She was like a bright light walking into the room. But underneath was so much fatigue and anxiety. Halfway through the session, she laughed uneasily and said to me, "I am the most boring person in the world. After seven p.m., I have to do everything just right. Then maybe, just maybe, I will be able to fall asleep."

The anxious type will have trouble falling asleep from one hour to a good couple of hours.

A second scenario for the anxious type is where the person may or may not have trouble falling asleep, but they wake up around 2 or 3 a.m., possibly even later, and have a light sleep for the rest of the night. My patients say they don't sleep after that time, but after questioning them a little more, they admit that they do. However, the sleep lacks quality. It's choppy and unrestful.

Characteristics of the anxious insomniac

Anna is certainly typical for the anxious type who cannot initiate sleep. But she was also aware of what could make a difference. What made her "the most boring person in the world" was her realization that a very long wind-down process could potentially help her fall asleep. So starting around seven o'clock, when her daughter went to bed, she would take a hot bath, prepare her bedroom, brush her teeth, and read for a long time.

She could not be with her husband in the evenings as any kind of conversation would be too stimulating. She would never take any phone calls after seven o'clock either, to the exasperation of her parents. Going out with her friends in the evening was out of the question.

The anxious type shows up in two different ways: difficulty falling asleep and waking up too early in the morning, with most people experiencing one or the other. Most commonly, this type presents with trouble falling asleep.

Here are characteristics of the anxious type:

- Unable to fall asleep for up to a couple of hours, though sometimes can be longer.
- More often present in women than men.
- Women in their twenties, thirties, and forties.
- Tired, but not groggy; feeling exhausted and somehow wide awake at the same time.
- Drowsy while reading, but as soon as they put the book down and turn off the light, they feel wide awake again.
- Anxious, unsettled; most anxious about the sleep itself rather than other issues in life. The following type, the overthinking type, may also have trouble falling asleep, but the anxiety shows up differently, as you will see in the next chapter.
- Easily excitable; good news, bad news, it doesn't matter; it is all stimulating news for this type as any excitement puts them on edge.
- Experiencing palpitations, usually with no medical explanation when checked, but seemingly associated with anxiety.
- Waking up after a few minutes of sleep, startled awake.
- Worse off before the menstrual cycle starts, though this hormonal connection is more apparent in the overthinking and overtaxed type.

Based on my clinical experience, the second variety of insomnia that the anxious type may experience is *early morning insomnia.* This variation of the anxious type is different than what Anna experienced.

Here are characteristics of the secondary anxious type:

- These insomniacs wake up too early in the morning, typically around three to 4 a.m. They tend to wake up gradually, in and out, not always even looking at the clock. This type of insomnia is common in both men and women.
- My patients typically describe the experience as: "I wake up a few hours too early and then I can't go back to sleep." Upon further questioning, they tell me that they do actually fall back asleep, but it's not good quality. It's choppy.
- The anxiety is not usually as intense as when a person can't fall asleep, but it's present; it's an angst sort of feeling, or a sense of dread, as you hover in and out of sleep. The sleep lacks quality and the person wakes up exhausted.
- This type of insomnia may be associated with sleep apnea. It's possible the sleep apnea episodes are more intense starting around two or three a.m.—the lung system time in Chinese Medicine—or simply that the nervous system is overwhelmed after repetitive stress from the lack of proper oxygen saturation leading up to that moment. Once the stress of those interrupted breathing episodes has been there for possibly hours, the body feels like there is a considerable threat and it won't go into a deep sleep.

Being in light sleep or waking up frequently in the wee hours of the morning is not normal, but I often remind my patients that we have more light and REM sleep in the morning than the first five hours of sleep, when deep sleep is prioritized. This reminder serves to ease off some of the anxiety that comes from the thought that we should be deep asleep and never aware of even one or two brief awakenings.

The anxious type with trouble falling asleep will feel more inclined to read something to help with falling asleep; the early-morning anxious insomniac will have no desire to pick up a book because she or he is feeling too groggy and out of it, unfocused and tired.

Some people develop both variations of anxious type insomnia, simultaneously. They cannot fall asleep initially and wake up too early. Or the insomnia troubles can go back and forth between these two, with patients having trouble falling asleep some nights and on others waking up too early. The overlap makes sense from my clinical practice, and it points toward the same type of dysregulation in the nervous system. Part II will highlight the root causes and how to heal these patterns.

The how and why of the anxious insomniac type

The anxious type does not develop trouble falling asleep overnight. If the insomnia is present consistently—a few nights a week, for example—it has been building for a while. In some cases, patients report that for some years they had a bad night here and there. For others, one day something just "snaps," and sleep is never the same. But again, even in those cases, the signs of imbalance were there; the person may not have been aware of the connections.

Intense emotional stress can cause this type of sleep pattern. A divorce, the death of a loved one, the loss of a job, or the birth of a child—though a happy event, it can be highly stressful, such as in Anna's case. If our body is resilient, we bounce right back. We may experience a few days or weeks of insomnia, but then we return to our normal sleep. However, if we have been stressed too much for extended periods of time, our body's ability to heal is depleted. The elastic is stretched for too long and it snaps.

"But then some people are stressed out of their minds for years," and they tell you they are "fine." You watch them breaking all the sleep rules, yet they never complain of sleep issues. That is because we are all born with different genetic makeups. We likely have also been exposed to various triggers throughout our lives, making us the people we are today. We all have strengths and weaknesses, and learning what they are helps us navigate where to focus. Those other people may be sleeping well, but their different health challenges will show up somewhere else if they keep up with a lifestyle that is less than ideal.

In Anna's case, she was stressed and had interrupted sleep for months. When her daughter finally started sleeping well, and through the night, her body learned there was a problem. So staying up was a protective mechanism. In fact, whenever emotional stress is present and causes insomnia, it is because the entire being is unconsciously staying up to protect itself or someone else.

For every insomniac patient who tells me they had insomnia since childhood, I know some childhood trauma changed their sleep patterns for the rest of their lives. In general, children are resilient, and even when genetic variants may contribute to developing insomnia, they still sleep well, as children and young adults, unless the nervous system was shocked to the core in some way.

This may mean trauma occurred in their life where the child felt unsafe due to abuse. But it may also be related to a "smaller" trauma. Somehow, they felt unsafe. Hence sleeping deeply was not a smart choice. When I explain this, many patients can pinpoint what may have caused the insomnia.

I have heard anything from moving houses, hearing parents yelling at each other at night, and alcoholic parents that neglected their kids, to being molested and always being on the watch because of it. Some don't know why, so shining a light on this aspect is helpful and can bring further healing through supportive therapies that usually include psychotherapy.

In Chinese medicine, the main axis of the nervous system is the heart and the kidneys. This axis is affected in the child who has experienced trauma. The heart represents the fire element, while the kidneys connect to the water element. They form a vertical axis, and the main idea is to keep each other in check, a healthy balance of water and fire.

This axis is the foundation of healthy emotions and sleep. Whatever that child subjectively experienced as traumatic and led them to have trouble sleeping—and when other signs and symptoms align with this diagnosis—I consider treating this heart and kidney disharmony pattern with acupuncture.

Another time when the anxious type's falling asleep problem may arise is in the late teens or early adulthood. Teenagers naturally want to go to sleep later at night. That is normal and usually reverses to sleeping earlier at night in their early twenties.

However, if the teens tend to push the time for falling asleep later and later, usually due to use of electronics, the body will have a difficulty adjusting to a more normal schedule. The young adult now may have to wake up early for college classes or a job. Some nights they sleep a couple of hours, followed by others, usually during the weekend, when they sleep for twelve hours or more until the afternoon. And so this erratic pattern develops. The person cannot consistently fall asleep at 10 to 11 p.m. to get enough sleep. Eventually, the anxiety starts developing, which may lead to long-term sleep struggles.

As far as developing trouble falling asleep or waking up early in the morning, the early to mid-thirties is a more common time for women to develop this dysregulation. The stress of the job, starting a family and caring for a young child, or a few, while working on relationship issues can all play a role in developing either trouble falling asleep or waking up early in the morning.

Perimenopause and suboptimal hormone levels can play a prominent role in this anxious type of insomnia. Women in their forties and fifties may develop insomnia for several reasons. Hormone levels shift gradually, which may lead to trouble initiating sleep or waking up early in the morning.

Surges of the stress hormone cortisol at inappropriate times, such as late evening, are also responsible for insomnia. Imbalanced cortisol levels are commonly seen in the anxious type. They get tired around 7 or 8 p.m., but it's too early to go to sleep. Then around nine or ten p.m., when it *is* time to go to sleep, the person will feel a surge of energy throughout the body.

Even though they are essentially tired, the rise of energy may feel like a wave of anxiety. Sometimes it can feel like an upward feeling from the belly to the chest. Others experience it like an intense buzzing or humming throughout the whole body.

Contributing to insomnia could also be a mismatch in sexual desires for the partners. Satisfying sex tends to lead to better sleep. Pent up desire or fending off an unwanted sexual advance because one is exhausted can lead to insomnia.

With hormonal levels dropping, a secondary problem arises. We lose muscle strength, including the tongue muscles and the muscles around the neck, and see an increase in snoring and possible sleep apnea. There may or may not be trouble falling asleep as well. Still, after sleeping for a few hours with multiple interruptions because of the apnea episodes, we may be wide awake around 2 or 3 a.m., experiencing the early morning insomnia we have discussed.

Therefore, it is essential to recognize the signs and symptoms associated with sleep apnea and then seek a sleep center to do a sleep study. According to the Mayo Clinic, some of the most common symptoms of sleep apnea are snoring, episodes in which you stop breathing, gasping for air during sleep, waking up with a dry mouth, morning headache, trouble staying asleep, excessive daytime sleepiness, and irritability (Mayo Clinic Staff 2023).

Men more commonly suffer from anxious type early morning insomnia. Their sleep starts lacking quality around 2 or 3 a.m. and continues until they fully wake up.

The four main categories causing early morning awakening insomnia in men are:

- anxiety due to stress
- sleep apnea
- frequent urination
- unmet sexual desires/needs

Healing the anxious type

It took Anna several months, but then the quality and length of her sleep gradually improved. About five or six months into the treatment, she came in and told me that she went up to the mountains for a few days with her friends. Altitude and sleeping in a hotel meant absolutely no sleep at all for her previously.

Yet this time something incredible happened. She felt like she was sleeping so well, she decided to have a glass of wine *and* some chocolate around 8 p.m. Her husband jokingly and apprehensively warned her not to push her limits. Apparently, he was a bit traumatized by all her suffering, so he feared she might get a flare-up.

However, she slept just fine that night. Of course, she is still mindful of her habits, and she tends to have her wine earlier in the evening, but for her to be able to change things up was wild and so healing. If you suffer from this type of insomnia, you know what I mean. Certain things that may be normal for some people may be a big, big no for you.

This type is typically more wound up. The busy person who never gets to slow down and always has an excuse not to slow down. This is the person who will exercise themselves to exhaustion and then realize this makes their trouble falling asleep worse rather than better.

If you have been around toddlers who skipped their naps for the day, you know what I mean. It's time to go to bed for the night, but they are too tired to even wind down and go to sleep. They are kids and still quite resilient, so after a few tantrums, they pass out. But you are so, so tired because you ran ten miles this morning, yet you are still awake and can't seem to be able to fall asleep.

The critical thing to remember is that we spend a lot of energy falling asleep and staying asleep. The brain spends roughly the same amount of energy when asleep as when awake (Richardson 2019).

When we are utterly exhausted, we can't even initiate sleep. You have to slow down physically to replenish. This is when I advise some of my patients to get in the habit of taking planned naps, most or every day. I know the advice around napping is controversial, but I have noticed in my clinical practice how napping can jumpstart the healing process for some of my patients. I cover more about naps in the sleep foundations chapter.

The healing of the anxious type can take time. The good news is that it comes with benefits. By trying to heal your sleep, so much more will heal. You learn more about yourself, you learn to slow down, and you learn to focus on what is most important.

Lastly, you learn more about self-acceptance. Healing this type of insomnia requires you to work on the anxiety piece by soothing and supporting the nervous system. It takes nourishing practices that tell your body and mind you are all right; you are safe.

Regardless of whether the insomnia is due to stress, hormonal changes, or sleep apnea, this entire healing process is about healing the root cause so the body feels safe enough to drop into sleep and stay asleep deeply throughout the night.

The anxious type has these common characteristics:

- This type either has trouble falling asleep for a couple of hours or wakes up too early, half asleep, half awake. Anxiety is present in both variants, often caused by the sleep troubles that are present.
- A dysregulated nervous system, hormonal changes —both due to menstrual cycle and perimenopause or, for men, andropause—or sleep apnea can often be why the anxious type can't settle into a sound sleep.

Ways to heal the anxious type:

- Understand how your nervous system works and how to downregulate the stress response so you can fall asleep and stay asleep easier.
- Explore the hormones chapter to balance and replenish healthy reproductive hormone levels.
- Consider introducing daily short naps to help you sleep at night.
- Further explore the sleep foundations chapter for tools and techniques to soothe your nervous system.

CHAPTER THREE

THE OVERTHINKING TYPE

A thousand things to think about.

The overthinking insomniac will either worry about things when trying to sleep or simply find themselves stuck on a thought of no real importance. One of my patients with a toddler boy told me how she would wake up in the middle of the night with her son's favorite song on repeat in her head.

I know this may happen to all of us when hearing a song way too many times. But when it's 1:30 a.m., this type of repetitiveness is particularly disturbing. Or it could be something you said to someone, or didn't say, wondering what they thought, and being unable to let go of thinking about it.

This type of insomnia shows up in a few different ways. Most commonly, the person will wake up after a couple of hours of sleep, around 1 or 2 a.m., wide awake and unable to go back to sleep immediately. In the majority of cases, the person will fall back asleep within an hour or two or, in a best-case scenario, within thirty minutes. This is followed by another couple of hours of sleep until it's time to wake up for the day. In the worst of the worst cases, he or she may never go back to sleep. They feel absolutely exhausted or sometimes wired and tired.

Or this type of insomniac may flip-flop between waking up at 1 or 2 a.m. and being up for a while and waking up and never going back to sleep. The overthinking type tends to fall back asleep more often than not after a couple of hours. On those rough nights where they don't go back to sleep at all, their condition may look like the depleted type, though as you will learn later, that type of insomnia is different in spite of this similarity.

Mia was a school principal with lots of responsibilities. She absolutely loved her job and, in fact, didn't find it stressful in general, but when she woke up at 1:30 a.m. most nights, she did lots of problem-solving, whether she wanted to or not. That is common in the overthinking type.

The second way the overthinking type will present is trouble initiating sleep. This person will be different from the anxious type in several aspects. The two of them may seem like they overlap, which is true in some cases, but they have some fundamental differences.

When patients come in, they often have been suffering for months, years, even decades. Their body has learned this new routine and partially, they sleep poorly almost out of habit. People often say, "I can't remember the last time I slept through the night."

Characteristics of the overthinking insomniac

A few years ago, I went through a particularly stressful time in my life. Lots of work, lots of studying, and then a big exam. I have never really suffered from insomnia, except for a handful of nights spread throughout the years. While my job is to help others sleep better, I was blessed with good sleep. Up to that moment, I had woken up for years, night after night, feeling grateful in the morning for the good sleep.

When I went through this intense stress and then started waking up at 1:30 a.m. for a few nights, panic rushed through body. I told myself, *It's okay, Damiana, you know what to do. Also you know why you are experiencing this, and it's going to be alright.* Well, all the reassurances I gave myself during the day did nothing at night. While I call this type the *overthinking type*, there is a layer of anxiety within all types. It's inescapable. However, the anxiety feels different.

Mia was constantly thinking about her school and the various meetings, solving problems in her head and so on. For me, it was overthinking and worrying. I would wake up, wide awake and wired, and then my brain would start spinning out of control from one thought to another. Sooner or later, as a byproduct, the anxiety would kick in. Eventually, I would fall back asleep, utterly exhausted in the wee hours of the morning.

Here are characteristics of the overthinking type:

- Wakes up around midnight, 1, or 2 a.m., wide awake and aware of their environment.
- Actively thinks about work or random things.

- Worries a lot.
- Experiences the worry and angst as soon as they open their eyes; as wake up, they feel an abnormal awakeness or rush of energy.
- Can feel wide awake, but usually before even checking the time, they can tell it's a different kind of feeling and likely not even close to the time they usually wake up.
- Shows up in both men and women.
- Tends to be chronic in men once it starts.
- Appears in women around perimenopause and menopause; associated with hormonal fluctuations and symptoms including hot flashes and night sweats. The hormonal patterns will show up in a few different types of insomniacs, but overthinking is the most common.
- Can be worse one or two weeks before menstrual bleeding starts if there is a hormonal imbalance.
- Involves blood sugar fluctuations.
- Can be worse with alcohol consumption.
- Can be associated with digestive issues.

In Chinese medicine, digestion includes digesting both food and thoughts. When our digestive system has a less than optimal function we have trouble with both. When we overthink, we regurgitate our thoughts and try to digest them over and over again. We are not built to do this. This is especially hard when it's the middle of the night and we would rather be sleeping than thinking.

Waking up in the middle of the night can be considered normal. We can assume our ancestors slept in two chunks. They slept for a few hours, and then they woke up for an hour or so to check in for safety reasons, stoke the fire, be sexually intimate, and so on. Then they would go back to sleep.

If you wake up feeling peaceful and you enjoy an hour or so of being awake in the middle of the night, I see no reason to try and change it. However, the people I see don't enjoy it, and they don't feel well. So we try to help them heal—either so they sleep through, or if they wake up, they feel good and are able to enjoy a short meditation or other activity, despite the fact they are awake.

The overthinking type can show up with trouble falling asleep as well.

Here are characteristics of the secondary overthinking type:

- Trouble initiating sleep.
- As opposed to the anxious type having trouble initiating sleep, they will have no desire to read.
- They will feel *so* tired but unable to fall asleep.
- Another common manifestation is a need to toss and turn, flip and flop, being unable to find a comfortable way to lie in bed.
- Falling asleep my take a few hours, but then upon further questioning, I find out that actually they doze on and off. They check the time and realize they must have dozed because time passed a bit too fast.
- They tend to think a lot and process information, but as opposed to the 1 or 2 a.m. awakening time, their thinking is hazier and more unclear. They can't really keep those thoughts organized.

Another expression of this same type of insomnia is the person who goes to sleep and knows they are sleeping, but they are aware of being in a light sleep all night long. Overthinking and worrying are not quite as strong here as the person who wakes up in the middle of the night; however, the root is similar. I often see digestive issues connected to this pattern. One of the major connections between the gut and sleep, which we will explore in great detail in later chapters, is that 95 percent of the calming neurotransmitter serotonin is produced in the gut (Terry and Margolis 2017, 319-342). Serotonin is one of the major calming neurotransmitters.

In some cases, the trouble falling asleep will extend into the whole night. This is a terrible scenario, and people who struggle with this feel intensely sleep deprived. They swear they didn't sleep a wink, though sometimes they admit it's possible they may have dozed very lightly.

Another expression of this same type of insomnia is the person who goes to sleep and then knows they are sleeping, but they are aware of being in a light sleep all night long. They feel as if they process information and sort of solve problems while half asleep and half awake.

I have treated a few patients with the overthinking type of insomnia who have told me it all started after being given antibiotics for a bacterial infection, such as sinus infection. Antibiotics can be life-saving. However, I recommend practicing caution with taking them or using probiotics to replenish the gut microbiome since the gut health is crucial for healthy sleep.

If you experience the overthinking type of insomnia, addressing your digestion is crucial. Even if you don't have many digestive symptoms, that doesn't mean your gut and its connections to the brain are optimal. The next section will explore this a little; however, the digestion chapter will dive much deeper into this subject.

The how and why of the overthinking insomniac type

When my insomnia kicked in the way it did, I wasn't very surprised. In spite of my lack of gastrointestinal (GI) symptoms, I knew from the Chinese medicine perspective that my digestion always showed a weakness. We saw this by looking at my tongue and taking my pulse, which gives a great deal of information to trained individuals, especially acupuncturists.

Susceptibilities show up way before developing noticeable symptoms or a disease. Changes happen in the shape of the tongue, its color, and the color of the tongue coating (fur), which gives us information before we are sick enough to see it in tests. The same way with the pulse; it offers a wealth of information well beyond our heart rate.

Let me tell you a little more about my health journey so you can see how subtle imbalances can be. A few years ago I did a routine check on my thyroid and decided to look a little deeper since I have a strong family history of autoimmune thyroiditis called Hashimoto's disease. I felt good overall, so I was pretty sure the results would come back normal.

To my disbelief, the thyroid antibodies were significantly elevated; my body was attacking my thyroid as if it was the enemy. My other thyroid numbers (such as TSH, free T3 and free T4)—typically checked at most doctor's visits—were still normal. But that is the disease process. At some point something changed, and my body started attacking my thyroid. My thyroid kept compensating, so the thyroid numbers mentioned above were still managing to stay normal while the antibodies were elevated. The question then becomes, how long will the thyroid be able to compensate?

Seventy percent of the immune system is located in the gut (Cacho and Lum 2021, 149), so with any autoimmune disorders, we have to look at the gut health. I already knew I had some food sensitivities, but my symptoms were never gut-related. I would instead get a headache from eating certain foods, such as gluten-containing foods. The stool test I ran after I received my thyroid numbers showed I had a large *Blastocystis hominis* parasite growth, and a high *H. pylori* bacterial infection in my stomach. When I treated those two infections, my thyroid antibodies decreased to one-third of what they were within just a few short months. I can't say my digestion felt better since I didn't have many symptoms to begin with, but I realized I was more clear-minded than usual. That clearly meant I had foggy brain for so long I had forgotten what was normal!

The reason I'm telling you this story is because I often see this in my patients. When the overthinking insomnia type shows up, I suspect there may be some digestive issues. Some patients tell me they have always had gut issues; others will tell me they are not aware of any. We dig deeper for any signs of imbalances and treat them accordingly.

Regardless if a person has any known gut issues or not, almost everyone can benefit from an elimination diet. The elimination diet (also called the *oligoantigenic diet*) will eliminate some of the most common allergens such as dairy, gluten, soy, eggs, sugar-containing foods, and corn along with drinks such as caffeine, sugary drinks, and alcohol. We eliminate these foods and drinks for a month and then reintroduce them one by one and see if the body reacts negatively to any of them.

Most people react to one or more, and that is a good place to start healing the gut, even when we are not aware we had a problem to begin with. More about this and the many symptoms that may show us that there is a gut component to your insomnia will be covered in the digestion chapter.

The overthinking type of insomnia tends to develop over longer periods of time. Continuous poor diet and stress in our digestion will add up over the years, especially as we age and become a little less resilient. For example, studying intensely and over extended periods usually add new layers of stress, which will exacerbate the insomnia.

From the Chinese medicine perspective, all this new information has to be "digested" and stored in its appropriate spaces within our brain. Over and over again, I have noticed this to be true. When we diagnose within Chinese medicine parameters, we notice a weakness in the digestive area, but also we notice that the tongue becomes paler and more scalloped.

Some people may even become borderline anemic in these times of great mental need. A few years ago when I was going through my doctoral program, my health took a toll, and I noticed a significant change in my tongue color. From a healthy pale pink, it became noticeably pale.

People who tend to worry think it's their nature to worry, and they can't help themselves. The more stress they have in their lives, the worse it gets. Some of them will have OCD (obsessive-compulsive disorder) tendencies, or they simply try to control everything they can since so much feels like it's out of their control. Emotional stress is a main factor in this type.

For people who fall into this category, the overthinking and worrying comes first while anxiety is more secondary. For the anxious type, anxiety is more apparent and comes to the forefront faster. Of course, they too worry and fret.

But when they develop insomnia, it shows up differently in the body.

Repressed anger and deep frustration tend to show up in this type. The stress of continuous thinking, going back and forth, and the inability to speak up literally affect the microbiome. Interestingly enough, in Chinese medicine, when the stress system gets highly activated, as it relates to unprocessed frustration, it will affect digestion. The Chinese knew this thousands of years ago. Back then it might not have been about traffic frustration, I assume. But when it comes to unfulfilled relationships, I bet it wasn't all that much different.

Since the overthinking type is common in perimenopause and menopause, I believe long-term gut weakness will then affect sleep in combination with hormone fluctuations. The strong gut-hormone connection is mainly covered in the hormone chapter.

Just like with the anxious type, there are genetic components to each of the patterns we tend to develop. We are born with strengths and weaknesses, and as we move through life, they serve as our teachers. We all have some sort of challenges when it comes to what we were born with. So we need to look at how to get to know ourselves and always be mindful of what is important to address when it comes to health and well-being.

Healing the overthinking type

What helped Mia heal was first acknowledging that she had no real boundaries when it came to her sleep. She kept saying how she loved her job so much, and she didn't mind thinking about it in the middle of the night while she was up. Yet she hated being awake for a couple of hours most nights. I told her I too love my job, but I am not my job, and I have the right and owe it to myself and my family to live a well-rounded life. That meant leaving work at work as much as possible. Because of that, I would be a better healer and she would be a better principal.

Besides acupuncture, herbs, and some other recommendations, we decided to do something about those thoughts. I told her about a time when my mind was just as busy as hers, years ago when I opened my clinic. My mind was filled with thoughts, just like she was describing. We just couldn't help ourselves. One thought after another, solving a problem in our head, then on to the next one.

So I told her to do what I did back then. When I got home from work around 5 or 6 p.m., every time I had a thought, a task that needed attention the next day, or a worry, I would write them all down on a notepad I kept handy. By the end of the evening, I had emptied my mind. Then every time I had a thought that was already on that paper, be it later or in the middle of the night, I would simply tell my mind, *It's on that piece of paper and I will deal with it tomorrow.* Mia did the same, and even though she still woke up briefly in the middle of the night, she would easily go back to sleep.

For the large majority of patients with the overthinking insomnia type, it takes a bit of work to heal. Since we are often talking about the gut, diet changes are important. Those changes take time to make a difference in your health and it takes some amount of commitment to actually keep up with them.

Healing the gut entails more than just working on your diet, though that is certainly the best foundation. It takes looking at the health of the microbiome followed by the production of digestive enzymes, and so on, which is amply covered in the digestion chapter.

That was clear in my case. I ate very well, mostly organic and at home, no gluten, dairy, or eggs—the foods that were an issue for me. Yet, my immune system was too weak to tackle the large parasite population in my intestines and the bacterial load in my stomach lining. Taking herbs and a short-term round of medication helped eliminate these issues. As a result, the thyroid antibodies dropped within a short period, which showed me that the parasite overgrowth was indeed an issue for my body since nothing made much of a difference previously in the thyroid antibodies numbers.

The bout of insomnia that came up for me during that exam was due to a digestive weakness that was rooted in my genes and due to years of eating foods that were not right for me, intense studying for way too long, followed by the extreme stress of the test. My body simply couldn't take it.

When I would wake up at 1:30 a.m. or so, I could just feel the intense stress and worry in my head. I couldn't stop thinking about the test questions that I thought I got wrong. The more that I ruminated the more awake I became. Then the anxiety kicked in, and then forget being able to sleep.

Eventually, around 4 a.m., I would start feeling groggy again and thankfully would get a few more hours. Fortunately, I had a couple of acupuncture sessions and some therapy along with less work and more fun things, and I started recovering within a couple of weeks before it started becoming a chronic issue.

Since waking up in the middle of the night can be related to hormonal imbalances, in that case, we address the hormones. If night sweats and hot flashes are present, the fluctuation in body temperature will automatically wake you up. Many women debate whether the hot flash woke them up or not since they tend to feel it about a minute after they awaken. I believe the hot flash wakes them up; the fluctuation in temperature just happens internally beforehand, and as it rises there is a slight delay until it is actually felt as a conscious rise of heat.

Healing the overthinking insomnia type takes a fair amount of commitment and time. The best part about working on healing this type of insomnia is that you are also working on the gut, which will naturally improve many other aspects of your overall health.

The overthinking type has these common characteristics:

- This type commonly has trouble staying asleep, typically up from 1 to 3 a.m. They are wide awake, worrying about various things.
- The second way this type can show up is trouble falling asleep, in and out of sleep, barely asleep, some worry and especially processing of information and being unable to drop into a deep sleep.
- Digestive weaknesses and hormonal changes are at the root of this type of insomnia along with a dysregulated nervous system.

Ways to heal the overthinking type:

- Work on healing the digestive system by improving your diet and diving deep into the digestive chapter; that chapter will show you where deficiencies and issues may surface.
- If you are a woman and have middle-of-the-night insomnia, explore the hormonal chapter to optimize your hormonal health.
- Explore the nervous system chapter to see how you can support a healthy, deep sleep.
- Look into creating healthy boundaries to deeply relax your nervous system at night.

CHAPTER FOUR

THE OVERTAXED TYPE

Always going, going, going.

The overtaxed insomniac type is the epitome of our society. We work hard, then even harder, and just when we think we can't do more, we push ourselves even farther. We may only stop when we become ill and the body forces us to listen. Men and women are equally guilty of not knowing how to balance work, play and rest.

I live in an area where the population is highly physically active. Almost to a fault. Andrew came in with insomnia that started about a year previously and gradually worsened. It began with his divorce, which was a long, drawn-out process, so he was actually happy when it was finalized.

He then decided to try and get in shape. He had little time during the day between his job and taking care of his two kids part time. He started to work out at 5 to 6 a.m. each morning, the only time he could find. He used to sleep soundly for years until 6 a.m., even through the stressful months of trying to finalize his divorce. So this was going to be a shift on his typical sleep and wake routine.

At first, he had a lot of trouble waking up at 5 a.m., but he did it anyway because when he made up his mind to do something, he would always follow through. A few weeks into his new workout, he noticed he started waking up before the alarm clock, by about thirty minutes. He felt wide awake and a bit wired but still tired.

Then, gradually, a few times a week he woke up at 3:30 a.m. or even 3 a.m. and was unable to go back to sleep. He tried all sorts of herbs and supplements but to no avail. Some nights he slept until close to his alarm. Others, he would be up at 3 or 4 a.m. This is the most typical pattern for the overtaxed type. Stress is the leading cause of this insomnia. Although stress, as you will see, plays a role in every insomnia type.

Characteristics of the overtaxed type

Andrew thought he was doing a good thing by waking up earlier in the morning, but his body was on edge and waking up earlier was perceived as a stressor, almost like a threat—a danger signal. His body was pushed to its limits.

Despite the stress over the previous months, he had had a good routine and his internal clock reliably knew that 6 a.m. was the wakeup time, which was a good thing. When Andrew moved his time earlier and then also exercised vigorously, he started developing insomnia, likely due to a stressed nervous system and abnormal cortisol response. This is just one scenario that leads to this sort of insomnia. More commonly, the intense daily stress exposure leads to these early morning awakenings.

He tried his best to understand what was going on. He was making better choices for himself, yet he couldn't sleep well, which started affecting his memory and concentration. He thought that by working out he would shed the extra fifteen pounds he'd gained over the previous years, yet he noticed he actually gained a few pounds. He started skipping some of his early morning workouts, thinking he just needed to sleep in, but it was a hit-or-miss situation.

Here are characteristics of the overtaxed type:

- Wakes up early in the morning, feeling wide awake yet tired.
- Wakes up as early as 2 a.m., but more commonly around 3 or 4 a.m. Or any earlier than your usual time also fits in this category. If you typically wake up at 6:30 and suddenly you start waking up around 5:30 or 5:45, it can point toward the overtaxed type.
- Can wake up almost abruptly, like being jerked out of sleep.
- May grind their teeth, which can be present in other insomnia types as well.
- Experiences an active mind, not necessarily worrying but thinking about various tasks.
- Generally more common in men; however, a fair number of women will also experience this type of insomnia.

This type of insomnia can show up when we stay up too late, are stressed, working, watching TV, on social media, etc. We fall asleep eventually because we are exhausted, but then we wake up too early in the morning.

Healthier individuals and younger adults will typically not have this type of insomnia. Teenagers or young adults may party most of the night and then be able to sleep in later in the morning or even to noon. As we advance in age, this tactic doesn't typically work very well. We either sleep to our regular time, or worse, we wake up earlier in those instances.

In Chinese medicine, the liver is responsible for processing all sorts of stress in the body, including emotional stress, hormonal detox, and more; hence this type of insomnia may be worse in women the week before the start of the menstrual cycle, more common in women in their thirties and forties.

I have occasionally experienced this type of insomnia, and it is always related to more stress than my body is able to cope with. If I am trying to finish a project and stay up too late, I get a second wind. I finish what I was working on and then lie in bed wide awake, trying to calm my system. Eventually, I do go to sleep, only to wake up early, tired and frustrated.

We typically sleep in ninety-minute cycles, so if you wake up within fifteen to thirty minutes before your alarm clock, I usually consider that a good thing; your body has learned your routine and likely is waking up before starting to go deeper into another sleep cycle. However, if you feel extremely exhausted, sleep may still be an issue for you, which may or may not be related to this insomnia type.

The how and why of the overtaxed insomniac type

Stress is an overused word in our society. It encompasses many different emotions and situations for which we use one socially acceptable term. Most people don't sit down over coffee and tell you they feel afraid and sad. We call it stress.

It's not acceptable or common to share and admit how frustrated—especially sad, angry, hurt, ashamed—we sometimes feel. Instead, we shove it inside and put the "stress" label on it. Or worse, we spill it out over our most loved ones. On top of it all, since we don't process these emotions and let them go, we develop insomnia. That in itself will make emotional stress worse since we sleep to process and compartmentalize emotions. I can't tell you how often I went to sleep upset about something and woke up after a good night's sleep feeling that the sleep took the edge off of what I was feeling badly about.

When younger, we tend to be more resilient. We could push our bodies with sleeping at odd times, partying all night, drinking too much, and still somehow be sleeping. For some of us who may have genetic variants closely related to sleep issues, insomnia may start in the teen years or as young adults. As I mentioned, if insomnia develops as a young child, the root cause is likely trauma or a safety issue. Or we may have been fortunate enough to have had good sleep as children and young adults. But as we get older, sleep becomes a problem.

The reality is we have jobs, we have families, and we have finances to think about. Or whatever worries us every day. Rest, siestas, and long vacations are rarely encouraged. We prize the busy, seemingly productive person who sleeps four to six hours per night and gets more and more done. Many of us have good reasons for this drive—the pressure to perform, to do something with purpose, to help others, and to help the planet. There's so much to do; why would you rest and how could one ever make time for an afternoon siesta?

In Andrew's case, the last straw after the long-term stress was waking up earlier to work out. His body was managing alright, but when he pushed himself to wake up earlier, his body perceived that as a problem. As stress builds within our system, the body will do whatever it can to piece together four to five hours of sleep.

This number of hours is the minimum necessary to live but not thrive because it is not enough to function for long or very well. Anything above that is the cherry on top of the cake. So if your system is on edge, it tries to protect you by sleeping *just* enough and waking up to be alert and be watchful the rest of the time.

I can think of several cases when insomnia started because the person needed to push their wake-up time, suddenly, after years of consistent sleep times. This transition to waking up earlier can be done, but it needs to be done gradually so the body can adjust. If we move the wake-up time by fifteen minutes every few nights, your body will learn and likely feel sleepier and quickly fall asleep a little earlier in the evening to make up for that time. If the transition is gradual, and you listen to your body, it can all be done. This is discussed further in the sleep foundations chapter.

Stress in this situation is broader than just emotional stress. It could be stress that the body perceives due to high inflammation. It could be stressed due to foods we consume that we are allergic to or sensitive to. It could be because we live in a toxic, moldy environment, and we are not even aware of it. It could be because we are in a toxic relationship. Stress could be present because we have ongoing, low-grade viral or bacterial infections in the gut or system-wide.

It could be that we have parasites, just like I did, which at night produce byproducts like ammonia, which are neurotransmitter disruptors. Or it could be the stress of irregular schedules or night-time shift work. So addressing the root cause of this stress will help you sleep better and decrease the chance of cortisol and norepinephrine spikes that can jolt you wide awake (Hirotsu, Tufik, and Andersen 2015, 143-152).

Healing the overtaxed insomniac type

Can you imagine ever saying you are bored? Most of us are so busy that the word *boredom* doesn't exist in our vocabulary. Or if it does exist, what do we do when we are bored? We reach for our devices to watch a movie, read something, or go on social media and endlessly scroll. We are spending, spending, spending energy. We empty the health bank account by constantly withdrawing. To be abundant in any area, we must put in more than we take out.

The healing of the overtaxed insomnia type takes mindfulness and some honest reassessing of our life. What is really important? What do we truly need? What are we doing out of habit or because we are running away from feeling our feelings?

Andrew felt sad. He still loved his wife and missed being a family and having his kids and wife around. He felt angry toward himself and everyone around him. He felt like he somehow failed. He didn't want to return to the way things were, but he realized he wished he could at least make peace with his wife. But all of this was too painful to really feel and admit to himself. So instead, he pushed himself harder. "I told myself, exercise is good for you, right?" Andrew said to me, deeply frustrated at his situation.

Yes, exercise is good but *not* at the expense of sleep. This type of insomniac can benefit from exercise in order to heal, as opposed to the depleted type, but it's imperative to allow sleep to be the priority and allow enough time in bed. For

Andrew, I did acupuncture to soothe his nervous system and recommended he temporarily eliminate the exercise. When his sleep started becoming more solid, we ensured he got seven and a half hours. He would go to bed a little past 10 p.m., be asleep by 10:30, and up around 6 a.m.

Many mornings, he woke up naturally right before his alarm clock. When this routine was solid and consistent a couple of months into the treatment, we started shifting his winding down and going to bed earlier by fifteen minutes, every few days. As many days as it took to make sure the body clock would adjust and his sleep was consistently seven and a half hours. The importance of this amount of time is covered in sleep foundations chapter. Eventually, his time shifted early enough—5:15 a.m. was his sweet spot—so he could sleep well and exercise in the morning for about forty-five minutes.

The overtaxed type eventually evolves into the depleted type if the person has a weaker constitution or if insomnia goes untreated for too long. When I ask my patients about their sleep history, they often tell me how it has shifted over the years. Staying on medications or supplements that don't address the root cause will also drive insomnia deeper. When people try to get off medications, insomnia can worsen. At first, we safely assume it may be because of the rebound effect and/or psychological addiction. But as time goes on and the body gets used to the new norm, we realize insomnia has shifted, sometimes for the worse, unfortunately.

I am writing this now during the COVID-19 pandemic. While I am terrified that people are suffering and dying, and many others are suffering because they cannot work or are in abusive environments, I also feel within myself and others a sense of relief. Finally, we stopped. Many of us stopped flying, growing, and pushing. Others are working harder than ever, such as hospital and medical personnel, teachers, and grocery workers. But most of us stopped. This came with the opportunity to do less and be more present. I can't help feeling a sense of great relief. I went out for groceries yesterday, and while I was driving on my street, within a few short feet I noticed a person biking peacefully on the left. Then saw a mom on the porch reading to her two young kids on the right, yet again on the left I saw an eight- or nine-year-old girl sitting on a white fence and playing her almost-larger-than-her guitar. I felt happy and I felt alive. No more empty houses while the streets are filled with cars coming and going.

We are finally taking a break. Hopefully this sort of forced stopping won't happen again. But I am confident we can learn something from it so that in the future, we can voluntarily make such choices. There is always some reason why we can't. Ultimately, we have to be honest and take a hard look at our lives.

We think we need this and that and the other thing, but honestly, we don't. We want peace and connection. Yes, we want food on our plates, shelter, and clean water. And we want access to good education. All else is a preference or likely a luxury. We have forgotten this. We live in our bubbles. We are constantly told what we need and who we are—on radio, TV, social media, commercials, by society, and by the movies. If you want to heal this type of insomnia and prevent going deeper into the depleted insomniac type, it's time to slow down.

In women, this type of insomnia may have a hormonal component, especially when we notice that insomnia gets worse in the second part of the cycle. However, it can be combined or overlap with the depleted type that also wakes up too early in the morning. The following section covers this in more detail. Ultimately, this type is about identifying what stresses the nervous system and providing relief. This will be explained especially in the stress response chapter in the healing section.

The overtaxed type has these common characteristics:

- This type wakes up too early in the morning, as early as 3 a.m., or anywhere from an hour or a couple of hours before the typical wake-up time.
- There is a sense of being wide awake, with various tasks running through the mind, tired but unable to easily go back to sleep.

Ways to heal the overtaxed type:

- Explore the nervous system chapter to help regulate it and communicate safety in order to stay asleep longer.
- Learn how to mitigate daily stress through tools found in the sleep foundations chapter.

CHAPTER FIVE

THE DEPLETED TYPE

In deep need of rest, nourishment, and self-care.

The thread that underlies the depleted type is not being able to maintain enough sleep. Joan was sixty-five years old when she came to see me. She told me it didn't matter what time she went to sleep; she always woke up about four hours later. She tried going to bed really late, for her, around midnight or 1 a.m., so maybe she would get so tired, perhaps she could sleep past that four-hour time. When that didn't work and felt like torture in the evening, she tried to go to sleep earlier than her 10 p.m. usual time. She tried 9 p.m. and even 8 p.m. She still woke up four hours later; if she was lucky, she would extend the window to five hours before being unable to go back to sleep.

With the first three types of insomnia described so far, we find more of a correlation with the time of the night. For example, for the overthinking type, no matter what time they go to sleep, they will wake up at almost the same time every night unless the time they go to sleep varies by a few hours or more.

The depleted type can only typically sleep a certain number of hours. A common characteristic is waking up after an exact number of hours, even when trying to shift the time to go to sleep earlier or later in the evening. It's almost as though the body doesn't have what it needs to maintain enough hours of sleep.

This type will wake up, night after night, wide awake. Although at times frustrating, the person will largely feel resigned. This may seem similar to the overtaxed type, but the overtaxed type usually wakes up after a few hours of sleep typically around the same time, feeling wired and awake, feels stressed overall and with a more intense awakening, such as being startled awake or jerked awake. For example, if the overtaxed type shifts their going to sleep time to earlier or later at night, it will typically either lengthen or shorten the amount of sleep they get.

Joan struggled with this for years and years. Strangely enough, she was not as exhausted as you would have expected to see. Most people in this situation are desperate for more sleep. One of the biggest worries is understanding the consequences of insufficient sleep, which usually drives sufferers to seek healing.

The depleted type has to build its internal resources, though they often appear to be fairly resilient to the lack of sleep. The treatments may take longer than for most insomniacs, and different kinds of approaches, combined, bring healing. While sleep hygiene is essential for all types, in this type it is a secondary priority.

Characteristics of the depleted type

If I could, I would hold the anxious type in a blanket and assure them gently, "You will be all right." I would caress the face of the overthinking type and look them in the eye and tell them, "It's okay. It's all good. It all works out. You don't have to worry." I would hold the overtaxed one's hand and tell them the world would be okay if they slowed down. In fact, they and the whole world would be better off if they did so. With the depleted type, I would wrap all of that in and gradually let it trickle inside their being so they could finally heal.

In this type of insomnia, I see the long-term combination of too much, too long, and too far. The neurotransmitters are by now so depleted, when I administer a urine test, the GABA and the serotonin are often low. These insomniacs often might not even relate to my description above because some of them are not even stressed anymore. They live a lovely, peaceful life. Yet, they can't sleep.

Genetics play a particularly strong role in this type of insomnia. For example, if the person has a COMT variant (see the online genetics chapter) sooner or later mood and sleep disorders will play a role in their sleep, usually when they get older and their bodies are a bit less resilient than at twenty.

Here are characteristics of the depleted type:

- Waking up after four or five hours of sleep, possibly six hours for some people, more commonly on the shorter side.

- Unable to go back to sleep; not necessarily as wired as the overtaxed type; and not groggy or half-asleep as the anxious type who wakes up early in the morning.
- Feeling a bodily sensation of being done with sleeping in a way, yet tired and incomplete.
- Not necessarily anxious or overthinking, but may have a fairly casually engaged mind, as in ready to get the day started.
- While the overtaxed type may experience more anger and frustration for being awake early, the depleted type is more commonly resigned. Present in people in their forties at the earliest, but a little more common in their fifties, and most widely seen in their sixties and later in life.

Since this type of insomnia shows up later in life when the body is less resilient and since it has likely developed over decades, insomnia may never resolve fully; however, most people are pretty happy even with partial improvement, even if they may not be able to get their seven and a half hours of sleep.

One of the changes that may happen in this type of insomniac is, as they heal, they may still wake up after five hours or so of sleep, but then they go back to sleep for a couple more hours in the wee hours of the morning.

Supplements and food choices ensure your body receives sufficient nutrients to support good health. This is crucial for healing this insomnia type. As mentioned before, proper sleep hygiene is important for all types, but in this type, it's secondary to replenishing the body's nutrients.

Another type of insomnia may seem similar to this pattern, but it actually belongs to the overthinking type. The individual wakes up at 1 or 2 a.m.; sometimes, they go back to sleep, but sometimes they don't. When they don't fall back asleep, the pattern looks like the depleted type. The depleted type is usually very predictable, always after five hours, more or less. The overthinking type may have an occasional night when they don't go back to sleep, but they usually do in the wee hours of the morning.

The how and why of the depleted insomniac type

In Romania, I grew up watching the elders go through this type of insomnia where the sleep cycles shortened. We don't understand precisely why it shortens. I remember one of my first speaking gigs on sleep at a retirement home and being asked why we sleep less. Do we not need it? God knows we need it. We are told incessantly that we need more of it to prevent the development of dementia.

Research shows how the brain "cleans" itself at night. Dr. Maiken Nedergaard, a professor of neurosurgery at the University of Rochester explained it this way: "You can think of it like having a house party. You can either entertain the guests or clean up the house, but you can't really do both at the same time" (Michaud 2013). So it is with the brain. It's either awake and taking care of all the functions that come with being awake, or asleep and cleaning up harmful proteins.

So why, then, does this happen? Why do we develop this sort of insomnia when we actually need sleep the most? It is simply one of the results of aging. The body isn't functioning as optimally as it did in the younger years.

We are born with some genes that are protective and others that are not. If you think about it, our body works amazingly, most of the time, most of our lives. Even when we have a health issue, over 90 percent of our body, perhaps even close to 100 percent, works well. However, when we are in a disease state, we notice it immediately. So if a couple of genes with variants can affect sleep as we get older or go through something stressful to the body, it's most likely that these will be affected.

We are so much more than our genes. In Chinese medicine, we learn on day one that everything is interconnected. As I have studied deep into functional medicine and researched sleep, I see the same thing as the Chinese did. This type of insomnia typically develops over a long time. Chronic gut infections affect the microbiome and brain chemistry over time. As the gut microbiome changes, so do the production of neurotransmitters such as serotonin, which helps promote good sleep.

In Chinese medicine, we talk about the duality of yin and yang, or better said, their interdependence. Yang represents day, activity, warmth, and fire. Yin represents night, rest, coolness, and water. The Chinese medicine doctors noticed thousands of years ago how the yin gets depleted as we grow older. We literally start drying up—sorry, but that is what happens basically—as we get older.

So when it comes to sleep, all the fluids nourishing our bodies—hormones such as estrogen and progesterone and neurotransmitters such as serotonin and GABA—become less abundant. These are some of the body's yin fluids from the Chinese medicine perspective. The good news is that in order to sleep, we don't need to have the same amount of these vital fluids as we did when we were twenty-five years old. We just need *enough* of them.

While it is common in older people, this insomniac type is present in younger people as well. Usually, some extreme event precipitated this in the young. It could be anything like having an accident, going through a divorce, having surgery, or taking medications that had intense side effects, and ever since things were never the same.

Another cause can be continued stress or exposure to an unknown toxin that gradually depleted the body. When I ask what caused their insomnia, many say they don't know. They didn't think anything in particular did. Upon more questioning, we often find what may have triggered it. At other times, we can't pinpoint the cause. Regardless of whether we know it or not, something happened in the body that led to being unable to sleep.

Healing the depleted type

One of my functional medicine teachers, Monique Class, family nurse practitioner, said something in one of her lectures that stayed with me: "We heal until we die." That was profound for me because I have worked so hard for so long to help heal my thyroid. If I could just lift this fogginess, if I could just bring those thyroid antibodies to normal... and so it went on and on. I thought if I do *x*, *y*, and *z*, all will be well, and I can go back to not having to do anything particular for my health, except eat healthy and exercise. Then I realized it never ends. Staying healthy takes some work. I made peace with the fact that healing is a process and to continue healing, I have to be at peace with where I am in each moment.

For years and years, I considered this type of insomnia one of the most difficult to heal. When healing didn't happen as fast as expected, I thought maybe I was missing something, not doing the right combination of therapies, or perhaps, I failed in some way.

Then I realized I was placing expectations on my patients' healing process and timelines regarding how fast healing should happen. I was doing a disservice to my patients. Healing takes time. It takes time to heal from any of the insomnia types. But it takes a little extra time for the depleted type. The good news as I see it is that the people who suffer from this type of insomnia don't feel as exhausted as the other types.

In fact, many of these patients come to me because they are scared about what science tells them not enough sleep can do to them. That is one of the main drivers. The other types are often worried, too; however, their fatigue and inability to function well is a greater issue.

Joan's insomnia improved over about a one-year period. The process was gradual, but thankfully she was patient with it. She didn't see much difference in the first few months as I did acupuncture and herbs, but her low back pain had improved so much, it gave her hope. Eventually, she noticed she started sleeping a little longer some nights. The trouble sleeping and waking up early was still present on and off, but she saw an improvement she hadn't seen in fifteen years.

For the depleted type, looking into gut health and checking neurotransmitter levels is important. In Chinese medicine, especially when using herbs, we treat these imbalances by diagnosing the main complaint differently. Rather than looking at individual symptoms, we always look at them together. If I were to analyze what herbs I use, I would say I am replenishing the neurotransmitter levels, improving their communication, and addressing the imbalance in the gut bacteria. In Chinese medical terms, I may say I am nourishing the yin, the healthy "fluids" in the body. I am drying the "damp" in the gut.

Damp is stagnation, a depletion of beneficial bacteria with an overgrowth of harmful bacteria and candida, fungal overgrowth. These Chinese medical terms may sound different, but we are talking about the same things; we are just using a different language. The Chinese didn't have the concepts we are now aware of, like neurotransmitters. But when I look at their descriptions—often using terms from nature, such as dampness—I can see that they knew what they were talking about.

The only problem nowadays is that we are used to quick fixes. I even had to reeducate myself repeatedly and remind myself that as much as I want everyone's sleep to improve in a couple of months—that in itself is not even fast enough for some—healing can take many months. It's a gradual process; as long as we keep at it, whatever ails you eventually gets better and better.

Healing of the depleted type also involves looking at the toxicity we have accumulated over the years in our bodies. We are generally very resilient and our bodies can put up with a lot. We can compensate for a long time, but it costs us. The depleted can often coexist with the overburdened type, which we will discuss next.

The energy powerhouse in our cells is called the mitochondria. The mitochondria are crucial for an incredible number of functions. They produce energy to keep us going every day, and to help us stay asleep and perform all the functions that happen at night. However, if there is any threat, such as a toxin, virus, bacteria, mold, and so on, the mitochondria are used for defense and way less for energy production. The connection will become more evident as you go through the next chapter.

The depleted type has these common characteristics:

- This type has trouble staying asleep past five or six hours.
- They feel some frustration, although not wired or agitated, yet feel done with sleep despite not sleeping enough hours.
- Most commonly present in later years, sixties or later.

Ways to heal the depleted type:

- Explore the nervous system chapter to address possible neurotransmitter deficiencies and a cortisol imbalance.
- Focus on optimizing your gut health by exploring the digestive system chapter.
- Work with a practitioner to get focused support and allow a few months of continuous care before deciding whether the changes you are making are helping.

CHAPTER SIX

THE OVERBURDENED TYPE

"Something feels off. Everything I try is not quite enough."

That is what the overburdened type will often say when they come in. They've taken this and that medication and supplement, tried this and that type of therapy. Even if they may get a little bit better, it doesn't seem like they are ever making real progress. The overburdened type has its own characteristics, but it can also share similarities with the other types of insomniacs.

The fundamental imbalance in this type of insomnia is that we don't have enough of what we need to function well, *and* we have too much of what we don't need. It almost feels like something "irritates" the system constantly due to a lack of alignment.

Mike came in because he felt constantly tired and unable to sleep well at night. He accumulated enough hours, but the sleep was such poor quality he always felt exhausted the next day. He was a successful, forty-five-year-old businessman and his disturbed sleep gradually started affecting his performance at work. He felt that if this continued for much longer, he would not be able to lead his company. He kept saying, "It's like something won't let me sleep."

Not everyone will come in and have that sort of insight, but when I hear my patients saying this, I sense something is at play beyond the daily stress, depleted resources, or some system imbalance, such as hormones or digestion. Of course, at this point, various systems are indeed affected, but then I start looking at their insomnia differently. If there is indeed an irritant or irritants, we must remove that first and then continue the healing process.

Characteristics of the overburdened type

The good news about this type is that once we identify what is aggravating the nervous system and causing insomnia, the healing process can begin. The more challenging part is figuring out what, precisely, the irritant is. Thankfully, we can look at the medical history and start the detective work. When there is an irritant, clues can tell us where it originates. When we accumulate enough clues, we can hone in on the possible causes and do further testing to confirm.

Before we dive deeper into this type, I would like to preface that many of the characteristics here may have sleep apnea at the root. Consult with your primary doctor to get a referral to a sleep center for a sleep study. If you are diagnosed with sleep apnea, your doctor will prescribe devices such as a CPAP (continuous positive airway pressure) machine or a mandibular device. Then you can look further to see if you can find ways to improve your health and sleep beyond these devices.

Let's get back to Mike. His insomnia started relatively abruptly two years previously. We tried to identify if anything had happened back then, but upon lots of questioning, it seemed like nothing was out of the ordinary. He was living in the same house, hadn't remodeled it, which can be a source of toxicity, hadn't traveled anywhere, had no particular illnesses, and had no additional stress during that period.

I looked at all his other symptoms but not much was going on, except he felt like his sleep was not deep enough and he felt so tired. His thyroid markers were within normal limits and he had done a sleep study, which came back as normal. His diet could use some improvement, but he never had any digestive symptoms, except his bowel movements were on the loose side.

But then, when I looked at his tongue, it was redder than normal and extra coated, which showed he indeed had a digestive imbalance, even though he showed no significant clinical symptoms. Of course, except for his insomnia, which can indeed be related to digestion because of the gut-brain connection.

I started treating him with Chinese herbs and acupuncture, and since the progress seemed slow and he had an appointment with a naturopath, I advised him to ask for a stool test. The stool test revealed an overgrowth of abnormal bacteria and mild to moderate yeast overgrowth. That correlated with what I previously observed of his tongue. These new findings could have also been the root of his insomnia since yeast is inflammatory, and inflammation can often lead to high cortisol, more in the stress response chapter.

A few more months passed, and his sleep and energy levels improved, but only by about 50 percent. Then through a fortuitous incident when something broke in his swamp cooler, he realized his swamp cooler, and house, had black mold. It took him several more months to heal between remediating the mold in the house and detoxing his body from the mold, but then he was able to finally sleep again.

This case shows the complicated story of various toxic exposures. I have since learned to look for toxins through testing if I find no other obvious explanation. They are often not easy to identify and time-consuming to heal. But we come out of it stronger, wiser, and know our bodies better than ever. And that is a blessing in itself.

Here are characteristics of the overburdened type:

- Restless sleep throughout the night, in and out, and unsure of how much sleep one really gets.
- Chronic insomnia that is less responsive to medications or herbs for sleep.
- You feel like you sleep all night but wake up exhausted in the morning.
- A certain restlessness; some people feel as if something pulls them out of sleep.
- Frequent vivid dreams, which may be disturbing.
- Teeth grinding, which is generally due to stress, but having a toxic environment is an internal stressor.
- Pain may be a factor that causes this type of insomnia.
- Often other chronic illnesses are present, though I have seen cases as exemplified above where insomnia is the main symptom.

- Digestive troubles and food sensitivities; food sensitivities can activate inflammatory markers leading to insomnia. Some of these patients notice that their insomnia is worse some nights, and not so much others, depending on what they ate.
- Chronic infections such as EBV (Epstein-Barr virus) and Lyme disease. These chronic infections and reactivations can be associated with various types of insomnia, depending on your susceptibility, but tend to play a more significant role in the overburdened type.
- Gut infections such as bacterial overgrowth (including *H. pylori*), fungal overgrowth (most commonly yeast), parasites, and worms.
- Sleep apnea; regardless of why it developed, the interrupted breathing will constantly pull you out of sleep and stress your body.

This is not an all-inclusive list, but it covers the main situations I see in my practice. Note that this type may show up by itself or in combination with one of the other insomnia types.

The how and why of the overburdened insomniac type

The overburdened type results from a society bombarded with less than healthy food, environmental toxins that include unhealthy products within our households, and chronic infections. All of these lead to inflammation. When we are inflamed, we are, in a sense, in a state of hyper-alertness (Liu et al. 2017, 316).

Some of us are blessed with good sleep, no matter how healthy or unhealthy our habits are. Others have been born with genes that, when expressed due to a less-than-ideal environment in our body, cause insomnia to arise.

Our bodies come equipped with an excellent detoxification system. However, when we have more toxins in the body than our detox system can efficiently eliminate, we accumulate what we call a toxic burden, which interferes with normal physiological functions and can often lead to chronic inflammation. Chronic inflammation, and elevated markers that result from it, can lead to insomnia. Viruses present in your body, such as EBV, can be reactivated and wreak havoc on your health.

We want to look at a few primary steps when regarding the overburdened type so we can understand how to approach healing this type of insomnia systematically. If you are unsure where the problem is, always start with the gut. Identify whether you have food sensitivities and allergies, check whether the gut microbiota is balanced, and finally, test whether there are any offenders such as parasites, worms, and viruses. If you are unsure where the problem is, always start with the gut.

The herbicides and pesticide exposure from our foods and outside environment may contribute to this toxic overload. Our mattress and bedroom environment can be a surprising source of toxicity. Our personal, cosmetic, and cleaning products are laden with chemicals; our liver struggles to clear them out of our bodies, and this less-than-ideal detoxification tends to affect various organs that eventually can affect your sleep.

Heavy metals are more and more prevalent in our bodies. Whether they come from foods, the environment, or dental work, they also increase our toxic load and can undoubtedly cause insomnia.

Mold exposure can cause many problems in our bodies, including stubborn insomnia, which can slow down the detox process and healing.

Regardless of where the toxic burden is coming from, it causes inflammation. Inflammation up-regulates the production of the stress hormone cortisol, and it negatively affects sleep.

Healing the overburdened type

The toxic load causing your insomnia may be coming from one primary source. But once your body is at a certain level of inflammation, it is wise to look at all the aspects of your life systematically. For Mike, insomnia led to discovering the black mold, which was revealed to be the root cause of health issues for his wife and one of his daughters. As hard as it was for him, he realized he and his family were much better off due to the many changes he made over the years since he started working on his insomnia.

He now understands how important it is for his house to be clean—free of mold, toxic cleaning product and personal products. He understood how his poor diet fed into the inflammation that was building in his body due to the constant mold exposure. We must create a clean environment at home, work, and in the car since we usually spend most of our time in these places on a daily basis. It is essential to ensure your bedroom is clean of toxins since we spend almost one-third of our lives in it.

Supporting the digestive system, regardless if it's directly affected, is of primary importance since this is one of the main ways we detox—by elimination. Regular bowel movements are crucial to detoxification.

Exercise and massage are important ways to encourage lymph drainage and ensure our kidneys and liver function well. Since so many toxins are water soluble, sweating is another critical way to assist the body in lightening the toxic load and start sleeping better. Sweating through exercise, hot yoga classes, or infrared sauna sessions will also support detoxification.

Using food to detox is the gentlest approach but also very effective if we stick to this way of eating long term since eating is something we do every day. In many situations, such as in Mike's case, we must add supplements or even medications. Since his mold markers were highly elevated, he chose an anti-fungal medication to start with followed by a regimen of supplements. The detox process has to be gradual; otherwise, you'll see side effects and might feel sicker than you felt before. The healing section of this book discusses this process more in-depth.

Healing the overburdened insomnia type may take time, but it will change your life and create a better terrain for your overall health for the rest of your life.

The overburdened type has these common characteristics:

- Restless sleep throughout the night, often feels like being pulled out of sleep
- Often less responsive to supplements or medications until the aggravating factor is removed
- Most common root causes: toxic overload, digestive troubles, chronic infections, or sleep apnea

Ways to heal the overburdened type:

- Identify what the source of toxic overload may be, remove it, and support the detoxifying pathways.
- Explore the toxic burden and chronic infections and biotoxins chapters to learn how you can support your healing process.
- Encourage the relaxation of your nervous system by checking out the stress response chapters.

PART II

THE STRESS RESPONSE AND HEALING

Part II speaks to the stress response and how it affects sleep. The first chapter focuses on understanding the stress response and its effects on sleep while the following chapter looks at the healing process.

CHAPTER SEVEN

THE STRESS RESPONSE IN INSOMNIA

Aim of this chapter

- Understand what stress is.
- Look at the various types of stress and how they might affect our life and sleep.
- Understand the cortisol connections in the body and sleep.
- Learn what neurotransmitters play a role in your sleep.

The effects of stressors on the body basically have no limits. The American Institute of Stress states that most doctor visits (about 75 to 90 percent) result from stress (2011). Chinese medicine concepts show no separation between the physical and the emotional body. Each organ, for example, is associated with a type of emotion or a spectrum of emotions.

Various ancient and modern thinkers believe an emotional blockage is the root of most diseases. When an emotional blockage or trauma is lodged in a particular part of the body, tissue, or organ, we are more susceptible to environmental toxins, poor diet, infections, and disease.

When we can't sleep, our bodies and minds are under stress to a certain degree; they are not entirely at peace. There is either too much of something, for example high cortisol at night or anxiety, or not enough of something, such as a crucial vitamin, like B6, or the calming neurotransmitter serotonin. Hence the body is literally under duress and cannot perform what is normal and desired at night—to sleep deeply and peacefully.

We have to look at the *whole* body to heal this innate stress response. How is the gut functioning? Are any pathogenic bacteria creating inflammation and affecting neurotransmitter levels to negatively impact sleep? Are the hormone levels not optimal and affecting neurotransmitters such as serotonin? The following chapters look deeply into these aspects.

Emotional stress is the first thought that pops into our minds when it comes to stress. Yet the stress mechanism is triggered by many factors besides emotional stress. It may be that your body is constantly overwhelmed with having to fight a chronic infection or bombarded with foods eaten daily that trigger an inflammatory response. That is also stress and causes the body to experience very similar reactions to emotional upset.

Emotional health is an extensive topic with multiple causes and multiple effects on your wellbeing. You may call it anxiety, anger, irritability, sadness, frustration, overwhelm, PTSD, trauma, depression, lack of motivation, withdrawal, etc. The combined painful and unwanted feelings are called *distress* instead of the more general term stress.

When there is emotional upset and turmoil, the psyche and body will feel the stress in one form or another. The emotional upset affects the nervous system first with bursts of epinephrine (also called adrenaline) almost instantaneously and cortisol within ten minutes of the initial stressor event.

Over more extended periods, stress affects the normal cycles of hormones circulating throughout the body. Many of my patients observe how their thoughts, time after time, take control of their experience when they can't sleep. It is rarer that someone is positive and peaceful when they can't sleep. Often I see frustration and anger. I also see shame: *Why can't I do better? Why do I let anxious thoughts take over? It must be my fault; I must be doing something wrong.*

Knowing our tendencies

Let's explore a few concepts about our tendencies as human beings to hopefully be able to position ourselves in a better place so anxiety and stress don't perpetuate and make our insomnia worse. And above all we must learn to be compassionate with ourselves and remember nothing is wrong with us, especially when we understand many psychological tendencies exist because of our human nature and our unique human experiences.

In the book, *A Clinical Guide to the Treatment of the Human Stress Response*, Everly, Lating, and Gravitz talk about a few eye-opening concepts, which hopefully will help you look differently at what your brain is doing at night when you can't sleep.

The first fascinating concept is that the brain tends to be more negative than positive. According to this book, it takes five to ten positives to combat one negative; therefore, one bad night and there we go, on a slippery slope that leads to anxiety and then more sleepless nights. The brain also tends to worry. The book says, "It acts like Teflon for good experiences and Velcro for negative experiences." What an analogy! If you are like me, I resonate with this so much. It takes time, effort, and practice to reverse that reaction eventually, but it is possible (Everly, Lating, and Gravitz 2019, 55-63).

Another critical concept to understand is that the brain doesn't like loneliness. Of course, everyone is different, and we desire more or less company; however, we generally look for human contact and companionship. It is tough to experience insomnia, as we are all alone, in the deep of the night, feeling like we are the only ones with this experience.

The doubtful brain is anxious and will try to fill in the gaps to find "an answer" to focus on as uncertainty is even more challenging. Regardless of what ideas pop up, they make us feel better than living in uncertainty. That's why thinking your insomnia is never going to get better is not the most constructive thought, but it can feel easier to deal with instead of just not knowing and feeling like hope is in vain anyway.

Our thoughts about our experiences can be changed and upgraded. Dr. Daniel Amen talks about this in a TEDxTalk: We are not stuck with the brain and mindset we have. Yes, neuropathways are formed, but they are constantly responding to new stimuli; therefore we can change those pathways (Amen 2013).

This book looks at various ways we can support this process.

Eustress versus distress

Before moving further, it is worth differentiating between the types of stress that we have explained so far and eustress. *Eustress* is a term coined by Hans Selye, a renowned Hungarian-Canadian endocrinologist, "eu" meaning good (Selye 1976, 15).

Exercising will cause more blood to pump through the veins; hence, one could call this stress—a need for higher activity and activation of various processes in the body. Eating creates a certain amount of demand, or stress, to produce proper digestive enzymes. It also triggers insulin production to keep blood sugar in check. An upbeat conversation may cause the body to create bursts of adrenaline and perhaps even cortisol. Still, as long as it stimulates healthy normal physiological activity or feels exciting and motivating, stress falls into the eustress category.

Generally, eustress is short term. It can be part of normal physiological processes because it enhances your capabilities and brings focus and excitement. Eustress fuels us to revisit a habit or hobby and be able to follow through. Without it, we would live in boredom. Ultimately, stress can be helpful at times but can also be harmful, and that is what we want to recognize going forward.

The problem arises when eustress crosses over to distress. If you are like me and many of my patients, we have been living in distress for so long that we don't even know what it means to live in a mainly relaxed or parasympathetic nervous system mode. Our lives are shaped by our upbringing, needs that come up throughout life, and demands dictated by survival. For the longest time, I thought I was the manager type who liked to start big things and juggle multiple tasks. In reality, that was my coping mechanism. Eventually, I realized that while I can have that multitasking mind, I don't thrive living it.

Stepping out of your usual environment helps you see your daily habits and tendencies. Vacations are great for this purpose. Not because one or two weeks a year will make up for all the stress you endured the rest of the time but because if the time away is long enough and peaceful enough, it will remind you of what is important and who you are at your core. Hopefully, with this increased awareness, you will gather the courage to change things when you return.

Otherwise, if you rely on vacations to get the needed rest, that won't happen. Three days after a break, you feel the same as before the holiday—yet again stressed.

Over time, we tend to adapt to stress since we are wired for survival. We get more sugar cravings due to cortisol surges, we produce more insulin to deal with the sugar, and then we store more fat. To the body, it feels like some greater danger is coming up, so we better prepare. With the insulin changes, sex hormone levels change as well. Reproduction is not as important during times of danger, so affecting the levels of your hormones is an excellent maladaptive mechanism. For example, if you are a woman in your thirties, juggling many things at work, and want to have a baby, your body won't know the difference between real danger or famine as opposed to daily chronic stress, and it might be harder to get pregnant.

The many layers of stress

Trauma, in a sense, is experiencing very intense emotional distress. The stress can be so fierce that it can make us physically sick within minutes, hours, or days. Yet stress goes beyond emotional stress.

There is physiological stress due to unhealthy diet. The body is overwhelmed with foods that it has a hard time digesting, which causes stress in the body. This is especially true when we eat foods that are highly processed with no real nutritional value. The liver needs to work hard to detox and then add the fact that your body is deprived of the necessary nutrients to thrive.

The body constantly needs to adjust and adapt to survive. It prioritizes certain processes—such as detoxing from chemicals, for example—and it neglects other processes, or at the very least they become secondary. That might not be evident to begin with, but after years and years of compensating, chronic disease arises. In fact, NASH (Non-alcohol related steatohepatitis) is becoming much more prevalent and is an example of a chronic disease brought on by an unhealthy diet.

Physiological stress also comes from bacterial, fungal, or chronic viral overload. The overgrowth of unhealthy bacteria in the gut competes with the beneficial bacteria. For example, overgrowth of the *Clostridioides* species, commonly found in the urine organic acid test I run in my practice, interferes with certain neurotransmitters and may affect sleep.

Parasites and fungal overgrowth, from *Candida* or mold, produce ammonia byproducts that elevate cortisol at night. Heavy metals burden the body and interfere with and inhibit specific processes in the body.

Chronic, prolonged exposure to daily stress will affect your nervous, hormonal, and digestive systems. It is just a matter of time before sleep challenges are experienced. Acute stress may or may not lead to insomnia, depending on various factors, including genetics. For example, it may start with an occasional bad night or a few nights a month, premenstrually. Then gradually, it gets worse and worse. For some people, the insomnia starts abruptly, with seemingly no explanation for why they can't sleep well any longer.

The connection between stress and sleep

Let's look at how the stress we experience daily can impact sleep. You start your morning by going to work. There, you are prompted by an email, a conversation, or simply because you are running late, and you feel stressed. That reaction may help you focus more, or you may find yourself tensing your shoulders and clenching your jaw either ever so lightly or more tightly.

Stress hormones secretion affects the digestive system, including blood sugar levels. Since the brain relies on steady blood sugar levels, hypoglycemia or hyperglycemia can cause insomnia. Also, sleep deprivation can cause elevated cortisol levels that lead to hyperglycemia, essentially an upward spiral that can lead to glucose intolerance or even type 2 diabetes. The body and psyche shift to deal with the threat by moving into fight or flight mode.

The stressful trigger signals the adrenals to release epinephrine and cortisol, and over more extended periods, the body lives in a constant state of hypervigilance, maintaining a level of alertness that does not allow for nighttime relaxation and sleep.

If you live in a hypervigilant state, such as from trauma and PTSD, any noise or movement at night will pull you right out of sleep in an effort to stay safe from possible danger.

Muscles tend to tense up with stress, and most people with chronic stress report tight shoulders and neck, clenching of the jaw, and teeth grinding. They also complain of being uncomfortable and unable to settle at night and go to sleep.

Stress can affect your breathing, and it can even show up as panic attacks in more extreme situations. In some cases, especially the anxious type, they can have a full-blown panic attack in the evening as they try to fall asleep or even upon waking during the night or in the morning. Once that stress response is unleashed, falling asleep is even more challenging. The stress may also appear as rapid, upper chest breathing and intermittent breath holding.

In the most extreme situations, you may be in such stressful moments that you have palpitations. At night, people report being hyperaware of their heartbeat as they put their heads on the pillow. Others feel their heart skipping a beat or two. This may also happen around 2 or 3 a.m., when they experience a blood sugar drop and wake up feeling the need to eat a snack.

Assessing to see if stress affects your sleep

If you have a sleep problem, it is safe to assume you have some stressor. The word *stressor* is used in a broad sense here. As emphasized in the previous section, the stressor could be emotional, a sugar imbalance, a pathogen constantly activating the immune system or a combination.

Lack of intimacy and support is a huge stressor. Grief and loss are also major stressors, and many people lost loved ones during the pandemic; certainly this has to be exacerbating sleep difficulties. If one becomes accustomed to sharing a bed and feels safer, it is a huge shift to sleep alone. This could be the loss of a human or even an animal companion. I have lost my dear Labrador retriever recently, and I know nothing can replace that gap in connection and comfort.

It is also safe to assume that our lives are never in a "perfect" environment. Our bodies have incredible abilities to adjust and even thrive in less-than-ideal conditions. For example, we may have a parasite in our body for many years, creating increased inflammation in the gut, yet live a thriving life. The fact that not all conditions have to be perfect is a beautiful thing. However, it is wise to question the status quo. A weak link may lead to another weak one; one day, more significant problems could surface.

Let's explore the various ways we can notice stress affecting us.

Insomnia as a stressor in itself

I wanted to start with this stressor because if you are already suffering from insomnia, this is important to talk about.

As sleepless nights creep in, the insomnia itself becomes a stressor. We build anxious thoughts around it, and it becomes a self-perpetuating negative cycle. The sleep deprivation will also negatively affect and stress your health. However, the purpose of this book is not to highlight the effects of sleep deprivation but to focus on natural solutions to support healthy sleep.

One of the signs that insomnia has become a stressor is that as the evening approaches, you start thinking about your sleep and get anxious, wondering if you will sleep tonight.

You also tend to hesitate to make plans in the evening or even morning out of fear that you may not be able to follow through because you may be too tired. This can happen regardless if that sort of issue was ever a problem.

Some people prepare excessively for sleep, wind down for hours, and feel anxious about any possible interruptions.

Or the opposite of the last scenario may happen. You avoid preparing for bed and winding down, instead staying up later to avoid going to bed out of fear that you may not sleep well.

Emotional and mental stress

As part of our daily life, we activate the stress response every day in a continuum that may range from intensely upset to living your days mostly at peace. We build conditioning within our bodies and hold memories in our tissues. This story would be different if we could start with a fresh slate every day. But every day, we build on the past. If you have a history of profound trauma, the rubber band snaps much more quickly. Building resilience helps our daily emotional wellness and sleep at night.

The large majority of insomniacs struggle with anxiety. The anxiety may have been present before insomnia kicked in or may have come due to sleep issues.

We have lost the confidence that we can quickly go to sleep. The mind makes up a story, and the body reacts. *I have been up for an hour; I only have three hours left. What if I can't go back to sleep like two nights ago?*

Biochemically, this stressful thought will send more adrenaline and cortisol rushing through the body. It is no different than waking up in the following scenario: at first not knowing why, maybe just an instinct, but then you realize a wild animal is outside lurking around. Of course, as a protective mechanism, your body produces cortisol and adrenaline to keep you up and deal with the threat. This wild animal scenario is no different than your stressful thought that you may not be going back to sleep, just like last week.

I have heard a great deal of worries and anxieties from my patients. You may feel resentful and frustrated about your situation, bitter toward people around you, resentful that you can't sleep while your partner may be plopping their head on the pillow and snoring the next moment.

Anger is another emotion I often see in my patients. You may feel this emotion toward people around you, family members, or even deceased relatives. We are usually *entitled* to feel anger toward someone who hurt us, but instead, we neither fully feel it nor let go of it. When we feel that anger deeply, we can move on. Buried feelings like this can keep us awake at night, regardless of whether we are conscious of these deep hurts.

Anger is a powerful emotion we don't give much credit to because we don't commonly encourage or approve of its expression in our society. But anger has energy; it has so much potential to move through us and help us heal. Many women struggle with the hormonal fluctuations throughout the month, but there is biological advantage to this.

These cycle fluctuations intensify emotions like anger and remind us what emotions we hold or push to the side without addressing. These fluctuations bring emotions quicker to the surface—for example, at ovulation or premenstrually.

Sadness is usually buried right under anger. Of course, sadness, or a feeling of being depressed, can be simply a result of not sleeping well. Physiologically, when we are sleep deprived, we don't feel excited about much of anything. From the survival perspective, this is a great coping mechanism. You feel apathetic, not up for anything, so it can be an excellent way to get the message to slow down and rest. In addition, when we suffer from chronic disease, sadness is often profoundly part of our identity.

Many people struggle with an inability to easily relax and experience a constant sense of urgency throughout most of the day and, unfortunately, at night too. They constantly need to do something, move around, be busy with something, take care of something, listen to something, or watch something. The reasons for feeling this way can vary, but emotionally, we are running from something. We are seeking a distraction from our thoughts and/or feelings, too afraid to stop and see what we feel. It's too much, too scary, or we have been doing this for so long that we don't know how to do it differently.

Anxiety may often take over your life, especially at night. One way to assess your stress and anxiety levels is by how you think about your day as you awaken and then rise. Is it filled with anxious and overwhelmed thoughts or looking forward to what the day brings? Do you fear that things will never get better or that your body may fail you?

Emotional stress can show up as constant negative thinking, such as worry, guilt, shame, self-criticism, self-loathing, and perfectionism. Or you may have underlying continuous stress about your home, work, and society roles. Or you may worry and have fears related to world affairs, the environment, and societal issues.

Some of my patients share having a sense of being out of control, like things are not real, basically dissociating from their bodies.

Another sign that it's hard to deal with emotional stressors is the need to keep busy in the evening with alcohol, movies, drugs, and so on; otherwise, the world feels like too much to deal with.

Some people have problematic relationships at home, especially with their bed partners; this is particularly important since we are physically close to them for about one-third of our day. Instead of letting go and being able to relax at night while in bed, as soon as we open our eyes, we remember our struggles.

You may experience a lack of emotional support from family and friends, which can be especially hard when suffering from chronic sleep issues. Or you may be afraid of being a burden despite having the support. Some people cannot accept help, slow down, or receive assistance when it is offered.

Lastly, emotional stress can show up as a lack of support regarding basic needs and a deep fear of not having enough to survive. Financial troubles that constantly make us feel like there is not enough to maintain support for our lifestyle and family, now and in the future, can be particularly stressful and disturbing to your emotional well-being and sleep.

Physical stress

I have briefly mentioned how physical stress affects the nervous system and can cause sleep problems. While I cover these issues in upcoming chapters, let's review some physical stressors.

Dietary stress can be due to food that has added chemicals, foods that we are sensitive and/or allergic to, foods that are highly processed and lack balanced nutrition, and foods that promote unstable blood sugar levels.

Poor water sources, dehydration, and ingesting highly processed or sugary drinks and caffeinated beverages can also create stress in your body.

Activation of your immune system due to acute or chronic infections, viral, bacterial, or fungal—examples: reactivated Epstein-Barr Virus, yeast overgrowth, and mold exposure—is stressful to your body. While this is a healthy and expected response, if the body resilience is low, poor sleep can result.

Environmental stressors and pollution from pesticides, herbicides, noise, electromagnetic fields, and toxins stress the nervous system.

Exposure and accumulation of heavy metals through foods, contaminated water, and dental amalgams burden the body. In addition, dental issues, including amalgams, periodontal disease that causes inflammation, and cavitation from infections in the root canals create more stress.

Other examples of physical stressors are acute or chronic pain that disturb sleep. The pain may be due to musculoskeletal stress and misalignment of the spine, or even intense physical labor or exercise.

Another common source of stress in the body is inadequate oxygen supply due to sleep apnea or a decline in lung function due to age or living at a high elevation.

On a more obvious side of stress and trauma, some people are in war zones or natural disaster zones such as people who have lost their home and community to fire, hurricanes, and even mass shootings.

The severity of the stress cannot be compared from one person to another because how we perceive it is subjective. One person may be able to sleep through intense periods of stress and even trauma while others can be easily triggered and be wide awake for hours and hours by the "smallest" trigger.

Spiritual stress

We don't talk much about this, but at the foundation of all stress lies our connection or the lack of connection with our spiritual roots. No matter what our beliefs are, most people believe in something, regardless of its name.

Someone once said that we forget our spiritual roots when we struggle with sleep. I would like to sit down and ask this person what she meant by this statement because, in my experience, the opposite happens. The purest essence within each one of us draws us to get to know ourselves better and look for a deeper spiritual meaning. They tend to pray more. Though I could see how, in moments of desperation, we lose our faith, entirely at a loss for what to do next.

Through chronic disease, we may experience a crisis in our values and what this experience called life means to us. I would argue that experiencing "dis-ease" may lead to growth and better things. But I realize not being able to sleep is hard, and the last thing most people want to hear about is the growth that will come from their struggle.

However, if we live in misalignment with our beliefs, struggling with sleep issues will force us to take a hard look and make changes. Everyone stands on the spiritual floor. So ask yourself, are your relationships, your work, and your life aligned with what is genuinely important to you?

Possible signs and symptoms of stress

We get used to who we have become, and unless somebody points it out, we are not even aware that our new normal is a stressed, always-on-edge kind of individual.

Here are some physical signs and symptoms that stress is affecting you:

- Rushing through eating. We all know that one! Or skipping meals because of lack of time or because you forget.
- You are being told you are a "type A."
- You find yourself clenching your teeth and/or your fists.
- You notice upper shoulder and neck tension or you feel tense muscles in general.
- You get frequent headaches, especially worse with work.
- You have a constricted throat sensation, or it's hard to swallow. Many of us find ourselves holding our breath, or it's shallow and constricted.
- You may also have clammy hands or cold hands and feet.
- Alternating loose stools and constipation is often a sign of stress affecting digestion.
- Concerns with high blood pressure, frequent colds and flu, loss of interest in sex, weight loss or gain, being aware

of your heartbeat, changes in your behavior (more addictive behaviors like smoking, drinking, use of devices).
- You may also find yourself jerking out of sleep after a few minutes of falling asleep; or waking up with a bad dream (night terror) within the first hour of falling asleep.
- You may have recurrent nightmares or disturbing dreams, restless sleep, sleep talking, or waking up in the middle of the night or early in the morning feeling wide awake, way before it's time to get up.

Diagnostic markers to assess how stress is affecting the body

My intention is to provide foundational details to increase your understanding of terms that are often thrown around but not completely understood or explained. I want to empower you. This is where we drop into the science a bit more.

How stress is affecting your body can be measured by assessing cortisol levels, adrenal function, and neurotransmitter function. Another disorder that can be tested is pyroluria, a genetic disorder that is exacerbated by stress. Pyroluria is further discussed in the online genetics chapter.

Cortisol, the stress response, and your sleep

One of the main ways stress affects sleep is via cortisol production. The adrenal glands, positioned on top of the kidneys, produce cortisol, a hormone that fuels action to find safety.

Cortisol has a few different functions, but in general, it is made in response to stress and danger and increases the body's sugar metabolism by breaking down glycogen stores and maintaining a set point of glucose that our body is accustomed to. If we are in trouble, we need quick and fast energy to help us, and glucose will do just that.

A healthy cortisol response spikes within thirty minutes of waking up to decrease significantly within an hour and then decreases gradually throughout the day until its lowest point at night. That's what gives you a wonderful *oomph* in the morning. It then drops gradually, especially after 2 p.m., and reaches a low point around 8 p.m. and for the duration of the night.

Chronic stress tends to disrupt this natural rhythm. We see this through salivary cortisol testing, looking at four to seven saliva samples in twenty-four hours. Many people who have insomnia will tell you that they can sense the abnormal shift; they understand what the reaction in the body is, and they can sense when it's happening. The cortisol levels rise higher than normal in the evening or at night, right when it's time to go to sleep. This cortisol curve then forms an unfortunate negative loop. We are tired during the day, wired at night, unable to fully sleep at night, tired again during the day, and so it goes.

Extreme imbalance in adrenal function and cortisol can result in Cushing's or Addison's disease. Cushing's disease is when the body produces very high amounts of cortisol, Addison's very little. Sometimes people have a pituitary adenoma or an adrenal gland tumor that is putting out high amounts of cortisol.

Over the next few pages I will explain more about how different cortisol imbalances express in our bodies. Bear with me as I explain the science behind this, as it will help you understand the next chapter easier when I offer solutions to heal.

When we find cortisol levels resulting in insomnia, we see an imbalance in the feedback mechanism from the hypothalamus and the pituitary—the HPA (hypothalamic-pituitary-adrenal) axis. Stress tells the hypothalamus to produce CRH (corticotropin-releasing hormone), which informs the pituitary to release ACTH (adrenocorticotrophic hormone), which then conveys the adrenals to produce cortisol. When enough cortisol is produced, the hypothalamus gets the message to stop production. However, if you live in constant stress, this cycle keeps repeating.

When the body reacts to a stressful event, the body produces cortisol in approximately ten minutes; what you feel first as a rush of energy through your body is the adrenaline rush, which kicks in within seconds and clears out of the body fairly fast if the "danger" or stress is brief.

In contrast, the half-life of cortisol is one to two hours. It is essential to understand this half-life of cortisol clearance because if and when we hit a second wind in the evening—likely a burst of cortisol—it will take time to fall asleep. So if you notice yourself getting sleepy, followed by being wide awake, give yourself time to get sleepy again. If you start having more anxious thoughts because you haven't fallen asleep within an hour, it will likely produce more stress hormones, including more cortisol.

According to research studies, many people with chronic insomnia may be in a constant hyperarousal mode during the day and at night, with a common spike in cortisol at night. The research also shows that factors contributing to insomnia are personality types that tend to overthink or ruminate, triggered by stressful events, and exacerbated by aging and the body's inability to adapt (Everly, Lating, and Gravitz 2019, 79-80). Yes, that answers why we could do anything at twenty years old and still sleep just fine, yet as we age, the slightest change can throw off our entire sleep schedule and rhythm.

Next, it is important to share the various cortisol imbalances. This information will serve as a foundation when I present solutions for cortisol imbalances.

Phase 1 cortisol imbalance

At first, when the body is in a constant state of stress, the cortisol may be too high all the time. That is Phase 1 of cortisol imbalance—*or circadian rhythm desynchronization of the HPA axis.* Whether we experience stress because of real or imagined dangers doesn't matter. The nervous system has the same activation of the sympathetic side.

Phase 2 cortisol imbalance

As the situation becomes chronic, the body chooses to no longer stay in constant hyperarousal and instead gives a spike of cortisol in the evening, when we want to go to sleep, to keep us up to deal with the perceived danger. That is Phase 2 of possible cortisol imbalance—*or paradoxical inhibition of the HPA axis.* This may also be due to a constitutional weakness rather than as a consequence or next step in this imbalance. Long-term stress also leads to decreased secretion of all hormones that are stimulated by the anterior pituitary. Manifestations of chronic high cortisol may also come in the form of depression, PTSD, chronic fatigue syndrome (CSF), or orthostatic hypotension.

Phase 3 cortisol imbalance

The third stage of possible cortisol issues is the uncoupling of the HPA and SA (sympathoadrenal) axis. There are two different pathways to respond to stress, both communicated from the brain to the adrenals: the epinephrine from one part of the adrenal glands, the cortisol from a different part of the adrenal glands. They usually act together.

Adrenaline gets produced very fast while cortisol is produced within ten minutes of a stressor. With the uncoupling of the HPA axis and SA axis, cortisol falls, showing decreased HPA function, while the SA axis is normal or even high. This imbalance is Phase 3 in the maladaptive stress response—the *exhaustion stage*. In this stage, there is a clinical picture of low cortisol and sympathetic nervous system activation of fight and flight.

This uncoupling may happen because the body still wants to respond to stress by producing epinephrine, but living in a high cortisol state is too damaging. The lower cortisol production is not necessarily a sign that the adrenals cannot make enough, but instead that they are choosing not to, in order to protect us from the high cortisol damaging effects on the body.

This constant state of *hypercortisolism* (high cortisol) has its own effects beyond insomnia. Such effects are related to functional hypothyroidism, hypogonadism, amenorrhea, metabolic syndrome, insulin resistance, abnormal lipid levels, hypertension, growth hormone suppression, neurotoxicity—affecting GABA, an inhibitory neurotransmitter, and glutamate, an excitatory neurotransmitter—hippocampal atrophy, impaired cognitive function, impaired memory, depression, osteoporosis, and immune system suppression.

This is why the body smartly shifts its mechanism in Phase 3 to a protective mechanism.

The cortisol awakening response

An essential layer of cortisol function is the *cortisol awakening response.* The cortisol awakening response is a normal physiological response to make you feel fully awake in the morning within twenty to thirty minutes of getting up. If it works well, you wake up refreshed and ready for your day.

The lowest amount of cortisol is produced in the middle of the night, toward the morning. In the last couple of hours of sleep, cortisol rises gently followed by that high spike within thirty minutes or so of getting out of bed. This is true for people who are not night-shift workers, in those people this pattern will be different depending on consistency of sleep and the times a person is sleeping.

If it takes an hour or two to feel awake, or you always need caffeine to get going, the cortisol awakening response is likely not working optimally. If you have a flattened response or even a downward spiral, you will have less energy, not feel as strong and healthy, and generally feel less resilient, physically and emotionally. You also have a higher risk of autoimmune disorders and a tendency toward mood disorders.

The cortisol awakening response is likely affected if you wake up and feel wide awake and anxious or go from zero to one hundred. If the response spikes too high, the stress response is typically easier to balance than when it doesn't spike. This response can be present in people with depression in the morning. One of the explanations why they are depressed is because high cortisol will stunt tryptophan's conversion to serotonin.

Cortisol is effectively tested with twenty-four-hour saliva testing. A one-time morning blood cortisol test is less valuable than testing saliva multiple times a day to assess the natural curve of cortisol. In addition, the blood test cannot assess the cortisol awakening response.

We have discussed how high cortisol harms our health. However, low cortisol levels, such as in the exhaustion stage, are also disruptive. Cortisol, in the right amounts, is highly anti-inflammatory, which is why we use prednisone, a synthetic corticosteroid medication, for pain and cortisone cream for skin conditions such as eczema.

Cortisol also helps regulate blood sugar and blood pressure and increases gastric acid production to aid digestion.

With low cortisol we may feel sluggish, slow, and as if we are trudging through molasses. Low levels of cortisol production can cause some of the following issues: pain, inflammation, allergies, low blood pressure, hypoglycemia, dizziness, lightheadedness, anxiety, more challenging time handling stress, insomnia, brain fog, low libido, and PMS symptoms.

Inhibitory neurotransmitters

The inhibitory neurotransmitters act as the brakes in the car—and the oil, I like to say. In balanced amounts, they calm you down, soothe you, keep you happy and content, and help you sleep well. Making GABA and serotonin depends on various factors, including gut health, proper nutrition, and genetics. Below are key concepts on how GABA and serotonin relate to sleep.

GABA (gamma-aminobutyric acid)

GABA stands for gamma-aminobutyric acid, a naturally occurring amino acid that acts as a neurotransmitter in the brain. Low GABA may show symptoms such as physical tension, unwanted thoughts, ruminating thoughts, or the need to self-medicate to feel calm, such as with alcohol.

GABA does not come directly from food but is a precursor of L-lysine and glutamate/glutamic acid, which is found in foods.

Foods rich in B complex are also helpful in producing GABA along with L-theanine, which is found in green tea.

Progesterone increases the effects of GABA, so it's essential to have adequate amounts of progesterone.

Serotonin

Serotonin is a chemical that nerve cells make, which sends signals between the nerves. Low serotonin can cause a busy mind, anxiety along with reprocessing, sugar cravings in the evening, PMS, hormonal imbalances, irritability, winter blues, impostor syndrome, and anger.

Ninety percent of serotonin is produced in the gut; therefore, gut health is crucial for serotonin production.

Serotonin comes from the amino acid tryptophan, which is found in food. However, tryptophan is less readily absorbable in foods high in protein because protein has other amino acids that compete with tryptophan's absorption. High-quality carbohydrate foods that contain tryptophan will deliver more as we'll see in the next chapter.

In addition, adequate levels of estrogen support serotonin production.

Melatonin

Melatonin is a hormone, but I've included it in this chapter because it is produced from serotonin. Melatonin is one of the most commonly used supplements to aid sleep. It is safe to use; however, it is only sometimes helpful since the cause of insomnia is not always melatonin deficiency.

Serotonin converts into melatonin in the pineal gland. This process requires sufficient serotonin and a functional pineal gland.

The pineal gland can become partially calcified, and its function may decrease. Causes of a partially calcified pineal gland are exposure to fluoride in the water and pesticides found in foods we eat.

Melatonin is also produced in the gut in a much higher quantity than in the pineal gland. Melatonin produced in the gut is an anti-inflammatory and considered a powerful antioxidant. However, the melatonin most useful to sleep comes from the pineal gland.

Iron is a necessary cofactor for melatonin production. Since women lose blood every month through their menstrual cycle, they are most affected by this. Check iron and ferritin (iron storage) levels to ensure they are optimal. While ferritin ranges are 10 to 120mcg/L, optimal ranges are between 70 to 110 mcg/l.

Melatonin activates the transition from T4 to T3—essential hormones produced by the thyroid.

Melatonin production decreases with age, so older individuals will likely benefit from supplementation.

Excitatory neurotransmitters

The excitatory neurotransmitters do what the name suggests—create an excitation in the brain. These excitatory neurotransmitters help with drive and focus but can also keep you up at night. We'll review the ones that relate to sleep next.

Norepinephrine and epinephrine

Norepinephrine, epinephrine, and a small amount of dopamine are produced by the adrenal glands in response to stress or danger. If you've ever gotten in a car accident or had a near miss, you know that feeling in your chest and belly of instant stress response. The adrenaline kicks in. Your attention is entirely focused, your body is completely engaged, and time seems to slow down.

To a lesser degree, this may happen throughout the day every day because of our constant state of stress. It can take milliseconds to produce these catecholamines, and if the stress is short lived, they clear out of our body pretty fast. While these neurotransmitters are excitatory by nature, either high or low levels can cause insomnia. Low levels will also cause low energy and lack of focus. Epinephrine levels are often elevated with ADHD (attention deficit hyperactivity disorder). Both MAO-A and COMT genes work on breaking down these neurotransmitters, so it's important to understand your genetic variants. More on these variants in the online genetics chapter.

Dopamine

Dopamine is the neurotransmitter that helps us keep focused, have drive and motivation, and be capable of finishing tasks. Medications for ADD/ADHD and caffeine aim to make more dopamine available. Dopamine is actually both inhibitory and excitatory. It is involved in regulating circadian rhythm and inhibits melatonin release through the pineal gland. Dopamine has receptors in the pineal gland.

Dopamine converts to norepinephrine through an enzyme called DBH (dopamine beta-hydroxylase) and with the help of vitamin C and copper. When dopamine builds up in the brain excessively, there is poor impulse control, anxiety, and developmental problems (Weiss and Marsh 2012).

Clostridioides bacteria in the gut can inhibit the DBH enzyme and stunt the conversion. Clostridioides is often elevated in patients' urine and associated with an imbalanced conversion from dopamine to norepinephrine. When insufficient dopamine converts to norepinephrine, they feel a lack of motivation and energy along with decreased mood. Reduced dopamine, on the other hand, can cause muscle spasms and has been linked to RLS (restless leg syndrome) and, therefore, sleeplessness.

Glutamate

Glutamate is a neurotransmitter that converts to GABA in the brain. If the conversion doesn't happen, partially because of gene variants, glutamate will build up in the brain, and GABA will be low, which is the perfect storm for insomnia—too much of an excitatory hormone and too little of the inhibitory and calming one. The bonus online genetics chapter covers more of the problem with the conversion.

L-glutamine is an amino acid commonly supplemented to help heal the gut lining. If you are experiencing more insomnia while taking L-glutamine, you may have an issue with converting to GABA and a possible build-up of glutamate. Glutamate will convert to GABA, but GABA can also convert to glutamate. It's like a two-way highway.

These will be the people who take GABA and aggravate their insomnia and anxiety. More about this in the online genetics chapter. Individuals with high glutamate tend to worry a lot and will have trouble falling asleep. They often suffer from anxiety and depression.

Histamine

Histamine is involved in the sleep-wake cycle. It is highest during the day and low at night. If you have trouble breaking down histamines, they can build up and cause insomnia. There is a natural release of histamines when we eat; therefore, eating later at night can affect some people.

Some sleep medications, such as Benadryl, contain antihistamines. Feeling groggy and sleepy is a common side effect of this type of medication.

High-histamine foods can be avoided if histamine intolerance is a problem. Individuals with variants in the DAO and HTNM genes, which are discussed in the online genetics chapter, can benefit from a low histamine diet and herbs to support the clearance of histamines from the body. The symptoms of histamine intolerance are discussed more at length in the genetics chapter.

L-phenylalanine

L-phenylalanine (PEA) is another excitatory neurotransmitter that gives attention and focus. However, there is an increased risk of sleepless nights if we have too much, mainly because it stimulates the HPA axis.

Elevated PEA may also cause anxiety and feeling over-stimulated. Low PEA has been correlated to ADHD.

Testing

Levels of these neurotransmitters can be assessed in urine tests. Various laboratories test neurotransmitter levels, such as ZRT Laboratories, Sanesco Health, and Doctor's Data. Organic acid tests and the DUTCH test have some partial neurotransmitter testing, though the first laboratories listed give a more complete picture.

Summary

- Stress can be present in our lives—from the insomnia itself to emotional, physical, and spiritual issues.
- Imbalance can drive sleepless nights, along with imbalanced excitatory and inhibitory neurotransmitters.
- The following chapter offers healing of the nervous system to encourage sleeping peacefully again.

CHAPTER EIGHT

HEALING YOUR STRESS RESPONSE

Aim of this chapter

- Learn and integrate the different rest types into your daily life.
- Learn steps to take when things are not functioning well in the body, such as looking at neurotransmitters.
- Explore foundational herbs, supplements, and therapies to relax the nervous system.

As you read this book, no matter which section you find yourself resonating with the most, take advantage of this chapter. Working on healing how your body responds to stress and building a more resilient nature within you is truly important.

The "Five *Rs*" (remove, replace, reinoculate, repair, rebalance) from the Institute for Functional Medicine is an elegant and effective way to approach healing. This five-step approach aims to heal the disease's root cause (Hanaway 2022). Originally a digestive approach, I have applied the framework to managing stress.

Remove

The absolute most crucial first step is to remove ourselves from the stressor. We can keep trying to heal our minds and bodies, but if you live in an abusive relationship, it will keep aggravating the wound. If we don't have enough resources to distance ourselves from the stressor, we start with more self-care so it may help us grow stronger and then gather the courage to take the next step.

The same goes for ongoing stressors at work and in our daily lives. Assess what exactly is happening that is causing constant stress and do not accept that there is no other way. I understand life can be challenging; we have responsibilities and things to juggle. Many times it just takes some willingness to be honest. Step back and take a look at your life, and sometimes you may need to make decisions that are scary to begin with.

If we live in a moldy house, no matter how much we try to heal the cortisol and inflammation response, we will never see enough progress if we don't remove the toxic exposure. The same with chronic infections, such as parasites or reactivated EBV. You have to remove the stressor or actively work on addressing it. The removing step also applies to foods that are not serving our health well, either because of their quality or our body's allergies or sensitivities.

Replace

The best way to build on *removing* is to *replace* what you just removed with something better. Years ago, I read this parable about a woman who lived in a house with ancient furniture. She had owned her furniture for decades, and it was truly falling apart. She had thought about getting new furnishings for years.

Since she'd struggled for years, she decided to get rid of it all at the same time. She placed all the furniture outside at the curb to be picked up in a few days. Then she sat in the empty living room, not having a place to sit or to eat but fully satisfied.

As happy as she was, she shortly realized that she hadn't planned how and when to get new furniture. The next time she glanced through the window, she longed for the old furniture; after all, it worked well enough.

This story is an analogy of our attempt to remove negative thoughts. If we don't replace them with positive thoughts, the negative ones will return fast. The same goes when removing foods that are not healthy. You have got to find a replacement, and you have to plan it.

With unhealthy relationships—be it work, personal, or family—when you make that incredible change, you have got to have the support lined up. In digestion, we add enzymes. We add healthier foods and ensure we can digest them properly. With a healthier stress response, we build our resources and become less reactive and more resilient.

Reinoculate

The initial inoculation of the gut microbiome happens as we are born through the vaginal canal. That healthy microbiota passes on from the mom to the child. We come into this world completely dependent on others, primarily our mothers. As we grow up as adults, as much as we want to take responsibility for who we are and our health, we are wired to need and help each other. This section discusses thinking about and looking for helpers in this world.

Assess what you tell yourself when you think about asking for help. It could be that you don't want to impose, that people won't help, or that you have gotten so used to doing it all on your own that you don't even know how to let others help you. Or you may have lost faith in the possibilities that open up when you ask for help, so you choose not to ask in order not to feel disappointed or hurt.

Another absolute primal need is the need for touch. Touch is the first sense developed in humans and communicates safety to us. Sleeping is all about having a sense of security and completely letting go, so we can peacefully drift away. The sleep foundations section talks about touch and how you can introduce more of it in your life.

Repair

Repairing is what you do after you get out of an unhealthy situation. You are settled into your new lifestyle, and you are now living just a bit less in hypervigilance mode. It is the therapy you do so you don't fall into the same relationships again. You build a new kind of resilience within your physical and emotional being.

You are healthy enough to start shedding what no longer serves you. Little by little, you repair the tiny, thousand cuts from many years of living this life. This stage is about tending to those scars. In Chinese medicine, scars cause blockages. Since the scars make you *you*, we don't want to remove them necessarily but rather soften them up so the energy can flow.

If you have infections in the body, this is the same step you do in the digestion chapter, repairing the lining of your gut. In this repair stage, we look at leaky gut (intestinal permeability) in digestion. With emotions, we can look at "leaky" boundaries in our lives and co-dependent relationships. These usually take much tending to heal.

Learning to say no is very important in the healing of your insomnia. Saying no may be tricky because you may feel like your livelihood depends on you saying yes. You might have said yes for so long that a relationship would become rocky if you started saying no now. However, relationships *can* rearrange and heal.

We need to improve at taking time between ends and new beginnings as a society. We are a culture of proud doers. We want it as soon as possible: the next job, the next partner, the next project. I am guilty of this, too. That space between ends and beginnings is called the *liminal space*. We are not very good at sitting in this space much because that would mean we would need to feel all the many feelings that we have been running from. It's easier to jump into the next thing. But the truth is we are tired, and we could benefit greatly from sitting in this space. Likely we would make better decisions moving forward that would improve our health.

Rebalance

Rebalancing is where we build stress-coping mechanism resources. We are increasing our resilience savings account for when stress gets more intense, such as losing a loved one, an illness, a breakup, or a car accident. We will still need time to recover and tend to these events, but the stressor can easily spin us into chronic insomnia and other health issues if we don't have some resilience.

The concept of "never well since," which is the existence of a trigger that came in at a certain point and caused health consequences from which you never really recovered, fits this scenario. However, if the health savings account had been there, it would have saved them from the down-spiral consequences. I see this with autoimmune issues where multiple factors come into play for the body to start attacking itself. The autoimmune mechanism develops over years and years. Then one day, something snaps, and we are officially diagnosed with some type of autoimmune disease.

One of the most important ways to build your savings account is sleeping. Since this book is for people who can't sleep well, I avoid discussing how sleep is so important. You likely already know. And you probably see the importance of sleep from all the various chapters related to the functioning body. But ultimately, we want to get to that better place and sleep well. Then get some more sleep. I tell many patients, "The more you sleep better, the more sleep happens. Once the body has all it needs to relax and maintain sleep, it craves peaceful sleep and will do anything to fulfill that need."

We want to achieve a place where everyday stressors are no longer overwhelming, finding a balance between not pushing yourself too much and learning to say no. We must be able to do things without second thoughts. You know what I mean by this. When we are sleep deprived, we can be super sensitive to everything. Every word we hear feels like a possible attack. A little injury or ache becomes an issue that won't heal easily.

The following section explores how we can encourage rest in our lives, probably the most essential gentle daily step to ensure better sleep.

The art of resting

Resting feels like a guilty pleasure if you are like many of my patients. Our society teaches us to be productive people. We demand so much of ourselves. After all, the world needs us; so many wrongs must be undone. And we want a fulfilled life. We want to accomplish something meaningful, and we have wounds that dictate our desires. Or maybe it's our most profound desires that dictate our life. Regardless of why we do what we do, resting can be easily labeled laziness.

We rely on vacations to recharge. It is unrealistic to think that a week or two here or there will give us the rest we need, especially when we also have trouble sleeping.

Even if we do sleep well, rest does not mean only sleep. Of course, sleeping is very restful. But what if you cannot sleep? And what if years of pushing yourself too much have led your body to stop sleeping well? As you know from this book, the answer is quite a bit more complicated.

Napping is one of the most remarkable ways to rest. It is particularly beneficial because it offers a break in the middle of the day. We have a natural dip in body core temperature, and even some melatonin is produced in the early afternoon.

We are meant for siestas. However, siestas are not part of our lifestyle, especially in the US. Try them over the weekend if you cannot nap during the week. The sleep foundations chapter goes into much more detail on why and how to nap.

In the book *Sacred Rest*, Dr. Saundra Dalton-Smith, an internist, shares seven types of rest: physical, mental, spiritual, emotional, sensory, social, and creative. Her book is wonderful and a breath of fresh air, so I highly recommend it. I think it would offer you more understanding and space to allow yourself more rest without guilt or shame (Dalton-Smith 2019, 5:26).

Insomnia rest

Before diving into the various types of rest, let's talk about how to take a rest from the insomnia stressor itself. Yes, we want to solve the root cause of insomnia, but after suffering from sleep issues for a while, the angst around it may also be a large part of the problem. Just thinking about the possible lousy night coming up feels like a full-time job for some people.

Here are some ideas on how to deal with this problem.

Think long term. I know it's hard because the effects of a bad night's sleep are immediate. Likely, the following day will be hard. But it's important to form some plan in your mind, take some actionable steps, and be able to tell yourself healing is gradual and will come soon. This way, you feel less pressure to "perform" each night.

We don't think clearly or all that well at night, so prepare during the day so you can rest in the evening and at night, even if sleep is not great. Think about how you'll prepare in the evening, what you will do if you wake up, and make it easy to do those things.

I know it's easier said than done, but every time you have a stressful thought about the coming night, let it go. You don't know what will happen tonight, and even if it's likely another insomnia night, you can do nothing about it right now. Unless you can do something, in which case, do that instead.

Listen to various meditations that help calm your nervous system, especially in the evening. Recordings that contain binaural beats can help you feel more at ease. Ask a therapist to help you calm down the anxiety. Watch your habits. Whether underpreparing or overpreparing for bed, see how you can make subtle changes that work for you and feel less stressful and angst-filled.

Emotional rest

Emotional rest is much, much needed, especially when suffering from sleep issues. The burden is often heavy, and it can get reactivated at night. When emotionally overwhelmed, all we want is a break, and sleep seems like could offer that respite. When sleep is not available, it feels even worse.

Some people feel dealing with a broken body is easier than emotions and trauma. However, we all must face hurt emotions sooner or later. Healing trauma is a process, and we are never done. Though some burdens are heavier than others, when we can let go, we heal our physical bodies by leaps and bounds.

Many of us live in an almost constant sympathetic mode. To heal our trauma and sleep, we must shift into living in the parasympathetic mode 80 to 90 percent of the time. With gradual relaxation, we can let the defenses down and rearrange how we function, emotionally and physically.

You can will yourself to take a physical or mental rest, but when it comes to emotional rest, it can be a little tricky. If your insomnia is emotionally draining, which it often is, until you get to sleep better, seek more support. The support can come from a good therapist, a spiritual counselor, a trusted friend, an acupuncturist, a holistic doctor, or likely a combination of these.

With insomnia, we might get our hopes up and be disappointed every night, so how do we protect ourselves against this emotional rollercoaster and get some rest? See the long-term vision. See if you can imagine a time when all will be better. See if you can roll with the ups and downs and remind yourself that even though healing is not linear, you are getting closer and closer to your insomnia healing. That sort of thinking can bring some emotional rest.

Suppose you sleep in the same bed with a partner you don't feel connected to emotionally or not as much as you'd like to. For now, one choice that would support your healing would be to consider sleeping in a different bedroom. Considering sleeping in separate beds can be a sensitive topic. Still, you can talk to your partner about your wakings and how you feel like sleeping in a different bed temporarily could help both of you sleep better. This temporary choice would allow you to be fully in your space at night and help you encourage relaxation.

For menstruating women, watch that week before your cycle and notice what emotions come up. Whatever you are feeling during that time is what lives deep within you. Yes, the hormones exacerbate those feelings. But if you feel irritated, angry, sad, and so on, those emotions likely live within you for the whole month. Take the opportunity to notice and give yourself grace.

The first few days of your menstrual cycle can be used as an "excuse" to slow down and rest. Slow down from doing, working, exercising, thinking, etc. Use your monthly cycle break to say, "I have no idea where life goes from here, but this is my time off to rest." Likely you will have to go along with whatever your life requires of you, especially with kids. However, anything that can wait, let it wait and do the unthinkable—be lazy. Of course, you are not being lazy, but I like to use that term because only then do my patients genuinely get it. If you are not feeling lazy, you are not resting enough!

Toxic relationships can affect us negatively, so surround yourself with people who leave you feeling happy, refreshed, and simply good.

Mental rest

Mental activity is much more tiring than we ever acknowledge with thoughts over thoughts and more thoughts. They are present throughout the day, and for some of us, at night. Overthinking or simply mental busyness is pervasive in many of us; trouble falling asleep or waking up in the middle of the night with ruminating is mainly present in the overthinking type.

We think tens of thousands of thoughts daily; unfortunately, many are negative. If you think about work and various tasks all the time and keep revisiting the same issues, it is helpful to start writing your thoughts down, especially after you get home from work. Keep adding thoughts, worries, tasks, etc., until the mind is mostly void of such thoughts.

Then when the mind revisits something you've written down, tell yourself, "It's written down. Tonight, I take a break, and tomorrow I will deal with them."

Multitasking can be very tiring mentally; we think we do more, but we become increasingly stressed and likely do less. Practice the Pomodoro technique, as explained in the physical rest section; these breaks will allow your mind to rest.

Some people struggle with mental fatigue more than others; hypothyroidism, mold toxicity, chronic infections, and anemia can all add to the mental fatigue of too much work and insufficient sleep. Unfortunately, the less we are capable of, the more we wish we could do just as we used to.

When you can't remember words or have difficulty concentrating, listen to your body, take it easy, and give your body a chance to recover. Remember that it is not random that you have a hard time performing; the body is slowing down on purpose so it can focus its energy on healing.

Physical rest

Physical rest encompasses more than sleep. Sleeping and napping are forms of passive rest, and we could benefit from active rest to calm down the nervous system. Some of my patients tend to overexercise, and make their sleep worse, feeling too tired to even fall asleep, especially troublesome for the anxious type. Good alternatives are walking gently, stretching, doing yin or restorative yoga, meditating, and practicing tai chi or Qi gong.

If you sit a lot for work, practicing the Pomodoro technique can allow you to move your body and offer some active rest in between. The Pomodoro technique is used for time and energy management to increase focus and productivity. You break up your work time this way: work for twenty-five minutes and take a five-minute break. Secret: That is precisely how I managed to focus and write this book. Take the time between sittings to walk around, stretch, take a few deep breaths, drink water, or make tea. Also, the time ratio between work and rest can be adjusted to meet your needs.

If you feel tension in your jaw, take a minute a few times a day to massage the jaw muscles, puff up your cheeks, and blow the air out gently; remember to consciously and consistently relax your forehead and all the muscles in your face. If you tend to build tension in your shoulders, take your hand, reach for the opposite shoulder, and grab that big muscle between the neck and shoulder joint. Hold and breathe for ten seconds; repeat three times. Then switch to the other side.

Napping can be considered active rest, at least partly. Every time I explain napping to my patients, I tell them that lying down in the middle of the day is not to nap necessarily but to rest. Just be sure to set a timer for twenty to thirty minutes to hold the space and so you can relax knowing if you fall asleep you won't miss something scheduled or important. More on this in later chapters.

Spiritual rest

Spiritual rest can be deeply comforting for many. Regardless of your beliefs, most people believe in something bigger than ourselves—something more than we can understand and more significant than this experience we call "life." So I ask all of my patients to find what offers them comfort and let that be the support when all else is too hard to deal with.

I recognize this truly may be uncharted waters for you as far as taking a leap of faith. Please read further to hear my thoughts on the nondenominational benefits.

Let your faith be the foundation so you can step into being hopeful and believing that what is needed for you to heal must be out there. When you feel so tired and broken that you don't think you can make it another day without good sleep, let that inner knowing that there is something bigger hold you and take you another step.

Surround yourself with people who share your spiritual beliefs so you can comfortably be yourself and rest from proving what you believe or having to fight with someone else's beliefs, which doesn't allow you to relax.

If you believe in prayer, however prayer may look for you, commit to praying every day for several days (seven, twenty-one, thirty, etc.) and ask: "I wish to heal and sleep well again. Let the right people, therapies, and situations show up in my life that will help me heal. I open my heart and mind to know that my sleep can heal despite the difficult truth of the past." Have some ritual, like being quiet in your prayer for five minutes every day, lighting a candle, or doing whatever else makes you feel supported.

Remember to love yourself and the ones you come in contact with. Love is universal. Practice compassion toward yourself and your sleep struggle.

Consider that most major religions have a weekly holy day for a reason. It's not monthly, not a vacation once in a while. It's a weekly day of rest. Ask yourself if you are truly resting that day?

Lastly, reach out to a spiritual counselor. They can help ease the heavy burden we carry when we can't sleep.

Adrenal and cortisol healing

Supporting the adrenal glands and cortisol production can be primarily accomplished by resting in combination with a diet that supports adrenal health, and herbs and supplements. The diet aspect is covered thoroughly in the next chapter, but I want to give you an intro regarding the adrenal glands and diet.

As a practitioner focusing on insomnia in my practice, one of the things I always check in with people about is the consumption of carbs. A few popular diets recommend a low-carbohydrate diet, but we need carbohydrates for sound sleep for several reasons.

First, a quick note on serotonin and carbs. We have to have enough tryptophan, which is found in the highest amounts in animal proteins. However, tryptophan is present in these foods along with other amino acids, which compete with tryptophan for absorption. Carbohydrate foods high in tryptophan offer greater absorption—more on this in the neurotransmitter section and the online genetics chapter.

Second, in times of stress, glycogen from the liver is depleted. Stores of glycogen are converted to glucose when in need. Sufficient glycogen stores are critical at night when fasting for nine to twelve hours. Those glycogen stores must be sufficient so your blood sugar doesn't drop and force you to wake up feeling uneasy, panicked, or even with palpitations in the middle of the night. This hypoglycemic state will activate cortisol production and aggravate the already malfunctioning HPA axis. That is why I don't encourage long-term ketogenic diets and rarely recommend them when trying to heal from insomnia.

Here are the steps to build a nourishing and replenishing diet to balance blood sugar and heal the cortisol response and nervous system.

Aim for balanced meals and snacks; we tend to include all three macronutrients (carbs, protein, and fat) in main meals but don't typically do so with snacks. Eating a diet balanced in macronutrients will help you sleep better and ease anxiety.

Drink a cup of water with lemon and one-eighth of a teaspoon of sea salt as soon as you wake up to encourage healthy adrenal function.

Eat within thirty to forty-five minutes of waking up to match the natural cortisol response. If the spike is abnormal because of HPA axis imbalance, this will encourage the healing of that natural spike. When eating, the adrenal glands produce cortisol to deal with glucose processing. If not hungry shortly after waking up, choose a smaller meal containing a small amount of fruit, collagen powder, ghee or half an avocado.

To heal your sleep, we focus on carbs from fruit and starchy root vegetables as opposed to favoring grains.

Tropical fruits (kiwi, pineapple, papaya) can be beneficial if consumed in small quantities and combined with protein and fat because they provide quick energy for your brain.

Root vegetables are high in vitamins and minerals such as magnesium, potassium, and vitamin C; they are complex carbohydrates that won't typically create a sugar rush, especially when combined with protein and fat. Root veggies can support serotonin production and, therefore, melatonin production. This is because root vegetables contain a good amount of fiber, which promotes healthy beneficial bacteria and, in turn, increases serotonin production.

Eat a small amount of fat with each meal; the fat sources can range from butter, ghee, coconut oil, olive oil, or avocado oil to fatty fish and grass-fed meats.

Eat dinner early, and you could try having a snack one hour before bedtime and see how it affects your sleep.

If you have been on a ketogenic diet, gradually introduce more carbs but not in the evening.

The "golden milk" drink can be an excellent nighttime snack. I have used this drink for years. Make golden milk powder by mixing four tablespoons of turmeric, two teaspoons of ginger, two teaspoons of cinnamon, one teaspoon of ground black pepper, and one-eighth teaspoon of nutmeg. Store it in jar. Use one teaspoon per drink. Mix the "golden milk" powder with your favorite heated milk like grass-fed milk, coconut milk, almond milk, or hemp milk, and one-fourth teaspoon of ghee, two tablespoons of collagen powder, and one-half teaspoon of honey. Another nighttime snack combines a small amount of fruit, such as half a banana, one kiwi, or half a cooked apple or pear, mixed with two tablespoons of collagen powder with water.

If you have HPA axis dysfunction, using caffeine to give you energy while also experiencing insomnia might not be the wisest choice. If you feel the need to have a cup of coffee, try "bulletproof coffee": six ounces of coffee, two ounces of almond milk or your preferred milk, one-half teaspoon of ghee, butter, or MCT oil (medium-chain triglycerides, found in oils like coconut), one teaspoon of collagen powder, and a pinch of ashwagandha. See more on this herb below.

Supplements for adrenal health

Using supplements to support a healthy stress response is a game-changer for many people. Talk to a trusted health care provider or pharmacist to make sure you have no contraindications. My intention is not to prescribe but to provide knowledge on what could be supportive for each individual with their current health and wellness regimen.

Take adrenal supplements within thirty minutes of waking up to follow the natural cortisol spike in the morning. They can be taken on an empty stomach. This practice applies to both herbs and adrenal glandulars.

Adaptogenic herbs help protect you from stressors; you could start with the adaptogenic herb ashwagandha (*Withania somnifera*) to support your sleep (Natural Medicines Comprehensive Database Consumer Version 2022). Some people, though rarely, react negatively to ashwagandha; one of the reasons may be that it belongs to the nightshade family, and some people are sensitive to this family. You could start taking ashwagandha in the morning within thirty minutes of waking up.

Phosphatidylserine is a component of our cell membranes and can help lower cortisol in the body. In theory, if you have high cortisol at night, the solution is to take phosphatidylserine in supplement form to lower cortisol so you can sleep.

There is one scenario when taking this supplement would be detrimental rather than beneficial and could aggravate your sleep issues. It is crucial to know whether your total output of cortisol is also high in addition to the free cortisol that may be giving you that evening rush. In this case, this supplement can be supportive. Work with a practitioner to see if this is right for you.

Phosphatidylserine needs sufficient magnesium to work correctly, so ensure you have adequate amounts of this mineral.

Licorice helps with cortisol balance by extending how long cortisol stays in your body, so this is only taken when cortisol is too low, and you feel tired. This herb can cause issues in higher dosages if you don't fully understand your cortisol curve and production.

In Chinese medicine, we use licorice in most formulas regardless of the complaint, in small dosages as a harmonizer, with no side effects. I am mentioning this herb because it is often found in adaptogenic formulas. Having the support of a practitioner will help you decide whether this herb is beneficial for you.

Other general adaptogens are rhodiola, which also helps with focus and memory, eleuthero, which supports the immune and hormonal system, and holy basil, which can reduce stress and anxiety.

Magnesium threonate, or Magnesium L-threonate, is the only type of magnesium that passes the blood-brain barrier and works best of the types of magnesium to help induce peaceful sleep. Magnesium glycinate is also beneficial to soothe anxiety and promote good sleep and is usually taken at bedtime.

Lastly, essential vitamins for adrenal health are B1 (thiamine), B5 (pantothenic acid) and C.

For a deeper dive into adrenal health healing I highly recommend the book *Adrenal Transformation Protocol: A 4-Week Plan to Release Stress Symptoms and Go from Surviving to Thriving*, by Dr. Izabella Wentz.

Neurotransmitter healing

Neurotransmitter balance for sleep is at the top of the list. Suppose you do not have enough calming neurotransmitters, such as GABA and serotonin, and/or too much of the excitatory ones, such as norepinephrine and glutamate. In that case, you will likely have trouble sleeping well.

If you've had sleep troubles for a while, you may have already tried taking GABA or even 5-hydroxytryptophan (5-HTP), a product of tryptophan that makes serotonin and melatonin. It may or may not have worked. If it did, you probably have to keep taking it to sleep well. There are ways to heal these deficient neurotransmitters in time, so you are not always dependent on these kinds of supplements to sleep.

To make these neurotransmitters, we need cofactors such as certain vitamins. Vitamin B6, particularly the activated form called pyridoxal 5'-phosphate, is required in the production of GABA and serotonin and often is found to be deficient in people with insomnia. Vitamin B6 and zinc also deplete in individuals suffering from pyroluria. Check out the online genetics chapter. People with vitamin B6 deficiency tend not to remember their dreams, but this is not universally true. Work with a practitioner knowledgeable with this disorder to safely take therapeutic dosages of vitamin B6, as excessive supplementation can cause toxicity.

B vitamins such as B9 and B12, along with SAMe (S-adenosyl-L-methionine), work in a complex dynamic through the methylation pathway. Supplementing with B9, even in methylated form, can backfire for some individuals, so work with a provider since you must take a few other steps before supplementing. SAMe is a necessary cofactor to make neurotransmitters. Check out the genetics chapter on my website for more information on methylation.

Over 90 percent of our serotonin is produced in the gut (stomach, small intestine, colon), hence working on healing your gut, decreasing inflammatory foods, and increasing healthy food that feed the beneficial microbiota is going help your sleep (Sjöstedt, Enander, and Isung 2021).

Certain probiotic strains such as Lactobacillus Brevis, Bifidobacterium dentium, and Lactobacillus Plantarum help produce both serotonin and GABA (Cheng et al. 2019, 632-648).

To support serotonin production we must eat foods that contain tryptophan and that are easy to absorb such as dates, papayas, or bananas. You could use a small quantity in the evening as your one-hour-before-sleep snack with some collagen and a little healthy fat, though you'll want to ensure the fruit quantity is small. Animal protein such as salmon and chicken contains high amounts of tryptophan, though not as absorbable but still beneficial. Oats, cheese, nuts and seeds also provide tryptophan.

Supplementing 5-HTP can be helpful in some individuals to increase serotonin. Tryptophan supplementation, which can increase serotonin in the brain, is not recommended since it can convert into a more neurotoxic pathway called the kynurenine pathway, which is inflammatory to the brain. Some individuals favor this pathway, even when not supplementing with tryptophan, as seen in organic acid urine tests or neurotransmitter tests.

Curcumin, the principal curcuminoid of turmeric, can decrease inflammation in people who favor the kynurenine pathway and is in general a great anti-inflammatory agent.

If you are taking SSRI medications and are considering 5-HTP, be aware of *serotonin syndrome*. You may try spacing out medications and supplementation. Talk to your doctor about this.

In addition, exposure to natural light, especially in the morning, encourages serotonin production and a healthy circadian rhythm.

Supplemental GABA can be used in the form of pharma GABA, which may be more usable by the body. GABA has a close relationship with glutamate. Glutamate converts into GABA, and it can go the other way, too. Glutamate is excitatory, so if too much is present in your brain, you will have trouble sleeping. That may also mean that GABA is too low, compounding the problem.

Rosmarinic acid helps prevent the conversion from GABA to glutamate. The standardized extract works best as it is more concentrated; however, you may try supplements or drink teas that contain spearmint (*Mentha spicata*), rosemary, or lemon balm. Spearmint contains the highest amount of rosmarinic acid among these herbs (Shekarchi et al. 2012, 37-41).

GABA is best taken in combination with L-theanine and rosmarinic acid. L-theanine is a calming amino acid that can help with both GABA and serotonin production; high amounts of L-theanine are found in green tea, so here is another reason to replace your coffee with green tea in the morning only.

Norepinephrine is one of the neurotransmitters that are crucial in the fight-and-flight response. Interesting to note is that benzodiazepines work by decreasing the firing of those norepinephrine neurons. One of the ways you can ensure that norepinephrine is better converted to epinephrine, and hence feel more relaxed, is by ensuring you have enough magnesium in your body as it helps this conversion.

High amounts of *Clostridioides* bacteria will inhibit the conversion of dopamine to norepinephrine. An organic acid test will confirm your levels. If a specific species of *Clostridioides difficile* is elevated, it is typically an emergency, as one symptom is bloody diarrhea. However, more negligible growth of *C. difficile* is not as symptomatic, though it can still affect the neurotransmitters negatively.

Healthy dopamine levels and conversion to norepinephrine rely on vitamin C and copper. Note that many people supplement with zinc for various reasons, which can, in time, tilt the ideal copper/zinc ratio, so testing is necessary to check levels when supplementing with either one. Vitamin C is required to convert dopamine to norepinephrine and helps calm the nervous system by decreasing the circulation of stress hormones. You may use liposomal Vitamin C as it stays in the body longer than other forms of vitamin C. Also, eat fruits high in vitamin C such as papaya and kiwi.

If you suspect histamine intolerance—a few possible symptoms are insomnia, headaches, hives, GI and sinus issues—check out the digestion and genetics chapters.

Melatonin can be helpful, especially in the aging population and for jet lag. A food that increases melatonin production is tart cherry concentrate. However, the concentrate is high in sugar, so I generally recommended supplements such as Herbatonin, from Symphony Natural Health, which is made with natural sources of melatonin.

Note that one side effect some people experience is vivid or disturbing dreams. If that is the case, melatonin may not be the best choice for you.

Since partial calcification of the pineal gland may be contributing to lower melatonin production, support your pineal gland health by using a fluoride filter to reduce fluoride exposure, eat organic to avoid pesticides, detox with supplements such as fulvic acid, curcumin, tamarind, and my favorite, raw cacao.

Acupuncture and Chinese medicine for healing

Acupuncture has been used for thousands of years to improve health, especially for stress relief. Stainless steel needles are inserted in strategic places in the body to help relax the nervous system and promote sleep. Acupuncture activates a communication system in the body that encourages your natural healing process.

Acupuncture increases melatonin production to decrease anxiety and increase the chance of falling asleep (Spence et al. 2004, 19-28). The amygdala (involved in feeling fear) shows decreased activation during acupuncture.

In a small study, acupuncture has been evaluated as comparable to the prescription sleep aid Ambien (Tu et al. 2012, 231-5). In another study, it has been shown to be more effective than Trazodone in the treatment of depression and insomnia (Luo et al. 2010, 899-903).

A systematic review of randomized trials on PTSD, which is often significant in people who can't sleep, and acupuncture has shown similar degrees of efficacy comparable to CBT (cognitive behavioral therapy) and SSRI medications (selective serotonin uptake inhibitors, such as trazodone) (Kim et al. 2013).

Acupuncture supports GABA production and use, may be supportive in cancer-related depression and insomnia, and may improve brain blood flow and have a tranquilizing effect (Feng et al. 2011, 199-202; Zhou et al. 2012, 302-7; Yan et al. 2010, 113-116).

Acupuncture sessions for insomnia are typically done once per week with a treatment protocol of twelve sessions. While each session may feel relaxing, it typically takes a few weeks to notice an improvement in your sleep.

Acupuncture is best combined with Chinese herbal medicine. Many herbs in Chinese medicine have been used for a very long time and have also been studied in scientific research. Chinese herbs are used at the advice of a Chinese medicine herbalist, who is almost always an acupuncturist, such as me.

Various other professionals may be instructed in certain types of acupuncture, usually for pain, but I recommend finding a licensed acupuncturist who treats internal medicine disorders, including insomnia and related symptoms. The National Certification Commission of Acupuncture and Oriental Medicine (NCCAOM) is the national board for acupuncturists in the US, where you can find licensed acupuncturists (nccaom.org).

Various other therapies and tools to explore

Many other therapies can help soothe and heal your nervous system. Some examples that have made a difference in my life and my patients' lives are somatic therapy, EMDR (eye movement desensitization and reprocessing), Brainspotting, Polyvagal therapy, guided breathwork, meditation, yoga, tai chi, and qi gong.

Step-by-step action items

- Take the time to observe yourself over a few days. Notice how you feel; when you feel relatively well and when you feel stressed. Take note of your symptoms and how they show up in your life.
- Take a piece of paper and follow the Five Rs (remove, replace, reinoculate, repair, rebalance): take your best guess or assessment for each category and write them down. For some of them, you can take action on your own; for some, you might consider the help of a professional.
- Start working with the basics. Regardless of whether you can sleep, you can start focusing on resting. Pick one or more of the rests and work on them gradually and systematically until you have covered them all.
- This chapter will be highly supported by the sleep foundations chapter, which will give you ideas on routines and how to treat yourself twenty-four/seven. If this is important to you, you may skip to that chapter and then return to the digestion and the following chapters.
- Look at your eating habits and follow the diet presented in this chapter. Adjust so it really works for you. For example, if a hearty breakfast works for you within forty-five minutes of waking up, great. If not, make a smoothie and make sure you include all the macronutrients.

- We have covered various supplements and herbs in this chapter. If you are unsure what supplements may be appropriate for you, work with a practitioner.
- Try a treatment course of acupuncture (typically ten to twelve weekly sessions). To get long-lasting results, you need at least a series and some maintenance (monthly or seasonally, depending on the amount of ongoing stress).

PART III

HEALING YOUR INSOMNIA

Part III looks at digestion, hormones, environmental toxins, and chronic infections—all as they relate to insomnia. As you dive into each of the healing chapters, it is best to understand the structure of each chapter.

Each healing chapter is broken down into several main sections. We look at the connections to sleep and why that topic is important in insomnia. For example, understanding the connection of the gut to sleep, or hormones to sleep, will help you better understand the correlations these systems might have for you when healing your insomnia.

Then we look at what signs and symptoms you may see if that system is involved and likely affecting your sleep. It includes laboratory tests you may wish to look into further with the help of a practitioner.

Lastly, we explore methods, tools, and techniques to start your healing process. You can do many of these things at home. This knowledge will affect your overall health as well since I am always aiming toward the root of the problem.

Always talk to your doctor, ask for help, and when needed, work with health care providers who are more holistic and understand an integrative approach to healing.

CHAPTER NINE

GASTROINTESTINAL SYSTEM

Aim of this chapter

- Understand what the digestive function is.
- Identify whether digestive issues may be present for you.
- Understand the vital connection between digestion, neurotransmitters, and sleep.
- Learn about the *Five Rs* of digestion and how they can change your life.
- Learn about the importance of healthy blood sugar for good sleep.
- Learn how the elimination diet is key to assessing for foods that are not right for you.
- Understand the usefulness of GI testing.
- Discover beneficial therapies to start healing your digestive system and your sleep.

When I first began writing this book, this was the first chapter. Then I realized that while the gut is critical, the stress response connects it all when we talk about sleep.

Healing your digestive system is an excellent place to start if you have obvious symptoms that relate to the gut. It is also the best place to start if you need help knowing where to begin the healing process besides working on the stress response, as previously discussed. As Hippocrates said, *"All disease begins in the gut."*

We can improve our health by focusing on digestive health and what we put in our bodies every day. We eat two to three times or more daily, so what we ingest is significant and can affect us positively or negatively.

Why digestion matters for sleeping

Before diving into the GI (gastrointestinal) system, it is essential to understand what it includes.

First, the GI tract starts at the mouth and ends at the anus. Various digestive organs are found mainly along this tract.

The digestive system is comprised of tube-like organs designed for transportation, movement, and absorption of nutrients through the body found along the digestive tract: mouth, esophagus, stomach, small intestine (which has three parts: duodenum, jejunum, ileum), large intestine (colon), and anus. The solid organs that aid digestion are the pancreas, liver, and gallbladder.

Neurotransmitters crucial for sleep are produced in the gut

Most neurotransmitters necessary for sleep (between 70 and 90 percent) are produced in the gut lining. The gut-brain connection is vital for a well-functioning nervous system conducive to good sleep and mood.

The gut is considered the second brain as it contains the enteric nervous system. The enteric nervous system is embedded in the gastrointestinal lining and can control gastrointestinal behaviors independently of the central nervous system. This is how a person with quadriplegia who can't breathe without assistance can still have functioning digestion.

Since there is a direct highway between the gut and the brain through the vagus nerve, whatever happens in the gut will affect the brain and the other way around. Hence, when your gut struggles with inflammation from an overgrowth of abnormal bacteria, low beneficial bacteria, or colonies of parasites, it will affect neurotransmitter production.

What is worse, the inflammation is sympathetic—fight and flight mode—activating and not ideal for good sleep. The other way around, when looking at TBI (traumatic brain injury), we observe the same phenomenon. Changes in the brain will affect the gut.

Inflammation in the gut produces stress hormones such as cortisol. While this is a normal physiological response, cortisol negatively impacts sleep and other functions.

For example, since the digestive tube starts at the mouth, oral health can significantly affect your sleep. We can see how this is true with how the inflammation from periodontal disease has been associated with insomnia (Tsuchiya et al. 2015,

83-90). Or in ulcerative colitis and Crohn's disease there is a negative loop between stress and the inflammatory response.

Since 70 percent of the immune system is located in the gut, it's essential to look at its health to keep in check viruses, bacteria, and any other toxins that may create inflammation in the body and lead to sleepless nights. Chronic infections will often lead to insomnia since they produce inflammatory markers.

Blood sugar regulation is crucial for good sleep and is one of the more common causes of insomnia. An inflammatory diet, including food sensitivities, can often be correlated to insomnia and hyperarousal because of inflammatory agents such as cytokines and prostaglandins.

Improper digestion of food connects to food sensitivities and a bigger chance of various damaging viruses and bacteria surviving in the body. With insufficient digestive enzymes, large food molecules will be present in the gut. The immune system will not recognize these as beneficial and will act as if they are a threat.

Also, with low stomach acid, more bacteria and viruses will thrive and make you feel unwell. Improper protein digestion will not provide the proper amino acids, such as tryptophan, which makes serotonin and melatonin.

Constipation assumes reabsorption of toxins and hormones meant to be eliminated while loose stools and/or diarrhea may lead to malabsorption of nutrients.

A low-nutrition diet will lead to deficiencies in important nutrients for sleep, such as magnesium, zinc, iron, and B vitamins. For example, B6 is a cofactor in converting L-tryptophan to serotonin and melatonin.

Assessing to see if your gut issues affect your sleep

Assessing for gut issues starts with noticing your body's signs and symptoms. Some will be more obvious than others. The trained eye can often spot imbalances before they become a more pressing problem. Functional stool tests through laboratories such as Diagnostic Solutions, Genova Diagnostics, Doctor's Data, Vibrant Wellness, and food sensitivity and allergy tests are often helpful in looking deeper into the function of your gut health.

Signs and symptoms you may experience when digestion affects your health and sleep

If you experience bloating after eating or a couple of hours later, discomfort, food simply sitting in your stomach, or a distended feeling in your belly or intestines, your digestion is less than optimal. Bloating can be connected with SIBO (small intestine bacterial overgrowth), insufficient digestive enzymes, or low stomach acid.

Feeling gassy should be rare with healthy digestion and absorption. We are told it's normal to feel gassy with certain foods, such as beans. However, if that is the case, it means the beans were not cooked correctly—i.e., soaking them for a couple of days—or you don't tolerate them well, and they are likely creating inflammation in your gut.

You may experience a painful sensation in the stomach area or intestines, the intensity varying from mild to severe, lasting from a few seconds to minutes or longer. If the pain lasts only a few minutes and is not bad, we tend not to address it. But that is a sign that something is off with your gut. Of course, we give it attention when it's more acute and somewhat painful. The go-to is often an upper endoscopy and a colonoscopy. If that comes back negative for any significant findings, we question if and what problem may be present.

A gnawing hunger sensation on an empty stomach, usually a couple of hours or longer after eating, could signal a possible *H. pylori* infection in the stomach, which is highly inflammatory to the body. While most of the human population has this bacterium in their stomachs, the growth and presence of active virulence factors are valuable information. Virulence shows the ability of bacteria to create damage in the body. Certain virulence factors are more health-damaging than others with some being strongly associated with stomach cancer.

Burping after meals can be related to low stomach acid production, subsequently a sign of incomplete protein digestion. In addition, low or normal stomach acid levels with a weak esophagus sphincter may cause acid reflux. Unfortunately, when that is the case, and we take acid blockers, we can cause further problems because of even lower stomach acid production.

Acid reflux is a fairly common symptom in our society, and it is often associated with allergies, food sensitivities, and an unbalanced amount of stomach acid. It can also directly affect sleep since it tends to happen at night when trying to fall asleep.

Adequate stomach acid levels are essential to protein digestion, assimilation, and keeping our gut microbiome balanced. The stomach acid will kill viruses and bacteria that would otherwise affect our body negatively. Proper amounts of stomach acid are also needed to produce vitamin B12.

Our bowel movements are not something we talk about often, but it's a helpful indicator of your digestive health.

Everyone is different, but generally, one to two bowel movements per day are ideal—formed, easy-to-pass stools that sink to the bottom of your toilet bowl.

Constipation can hint that magnesium may be deficient. Magnesium is the one of the most common minerals to support healthy sleep and moving your bowels. Less than one to two bowel movements per day signify slow motility. The concern with infrequent bowel movements is that certain toxins meant to be eliminated are being reabsorbed in the body.

Also, certain estrogen metabolites are intended to be eliminated in your stools. If they sit too long in your intestines, some will get reabsorbed and may lead to estrogen dominance. The balance and ratio between progesterone and estrogen as well as their effects on sleep are discussed in great detail in the hormone chapter.

The slow transit time and constipation may also be an indication of low thyroid function, imbalanced gut bacteria, or possible food sensitivities.

Loose stools come with their own set of possible problems—from imbalanced bacteria to food sensitivities and the danger of malabsorption of nutrients due to faster transit times.

Floating stools may be a sign of fat malabsorption. Sticky stools and the sensation of feeling unfinished when done with a bowel movement also signal improper digestion.

Of course, symptoms such as blood in the stool or pain while passing the stool are more pronounced, and we acknowledge more easily that something is amiss. Talk to your medical provider immediately if you see blood in your stool. Blood in the stool could be from something as benign as hemorrhoids or indicate more serious issues.

Some people get headaches after eating certain meals or simply suspect the headache may come from certain foods even if it doesn't come immediately after a meal. Unless you track those foods closely, it's hard to pinpoint if the headaches may be related to certain foods. Food sensitivities that trigger headaches or migraines can happen anywhere between a few hours to seventy-two hours from ingestion.

Something to consider is that migraine sufferers often have food sensitivities and/or allergies that trigger their headaches. In one study, 75 percent of women eating chocolate found a correlation to their migraines, mainly because of the Phenylethylamine content. Still, many other food correlations were found to trigger migraines, such as dairy products, tomatoes, some nuts, additives, cold-cut meats, alcoholic drinks, especially red wine, and many more (Nazari and Eghbali 2012, 65-71). I often see patients in my practice suffering from insomnia and migraines with food issues being the leading cause.

Sugar cravings are one of the most important aspects to address with sleep. Sugar cravings can mean our body, especially our brain, wants quick energy. The blood sugar imbalance may be present because we are not feeding it enough nutritious foods, or we have insulin sensitivity, and the blood sugar receptors have become less sensitive. We have two problems now. The bouts of *hypoglycemia* (low blood sugar), which can contribute to interrupted sleep, are likely rotating with *hyperglycemia* (high blood sugar), which is highly inflammatory and causes oxidative stress.

The brain depends on glucose. In the case of hypoglycemia, when glucose is not readily available, the brain will perceive that as stressful. Cortisol will be produced to help make more glucose available, and you will wake up in the middle of the night feeling wide awake. Similarly, in hyperglycemia, more cortisol will be present, which excites the nervous system and may lead to insomnia.

Gut immunity issues and candida overgrowth may be involved in recurrent yeast infections. Yeast is inflammatory and will create higher cortisol levels at inappropriate times, likely affecting your sleep (Kumamoto 2011, 386-91).

Immune and/or autoimmune issues *always* hint at gut issues since so much of the immune system is in the gut. If you have been diagnosed with an autoimmune disorder, the gut has been affected. According to Dr. Fassano—a world-renowned expert in celiac disease, intestinal permeability, and autoimmune disorders—to develop an autoimmune disorder one has to have a genetic predisposition, a gut imbalance, and a trigger like an infection, a car accident, an intense emotional stressor, or an exposure to a toxin or chemical (Fasano 2020).

Testing for digestive issues

Before looking at how we can test for GI issues, let's clarify why one test can't ever cover the complexity of this system. To properly assess the GI system, we are looking at three aspects:

Structural issues—scar tissue, polyps, rectal prolapse, damaged villi (finger-like projections in the small intestine) and gastro-esophageal prolapse (which can cause acid reflux).

Mechanical issues—chewing of food, absorption, and motility of the intestines (bowel movement frequency).

Physiological issues—production of certain substances, such as stomach acid, pancreatic enzymes, bile, CCK (cholecystokinin), immune function in the gut, beneficial bacteria levels, and overgrowth of bacteria.

Now you see why a colonoscopy can't give all the answers, as it primarily looks at structure. A combination of tests and assessments will provide a more complete picture of the health of your GI system. As a first step, always check whether a colonoscopy or endoscopy is recommended with your primary care provider.

A functional stool test will look at a variety of abnormal bacteria along with beneficial bacteria, parasites, worms, and digestive function markers such as elastase, which indicates pancreatic enzymes levels, intestinal health markers such as zonulin, which can show intestinal permeability issues, and secretory IgA levels, which assess immune system health.

The test for *H. pylori* is included in some stool tests. If not, a breath test is advised and is standard of care.

For food sensitivity testing, I prefer testing that looks at IgG but also further testing for the complement proteins, which lowers the chance of false positive. The elimination diet is the gold standard and highly recommended; however, food sensitivity testing can be quite valuable, especially when done in addition to the elimination diet.

Blood sugar testing includes fasting blood glucose, insulin, and HbA1c, which assesses your blood sugar over the past two to three months.

A SIBO (small intestine bacterial overgrowth) breath test will look at markers that indicate an overgrowth of bacteria in the small intestine. Bacteria should thrive in the colon but not in the small intestine.

Lastly, organic acid tests will give you a snapshot of many bodily functions, including digestive health.

Heal your gut and improve your sleep

Healing the gut is a step-by-step process. One of the first approaches to identify the root problem of your gut issues and forming a treatment plan involves the "Five *Rs*":

Remove: This means removing any factors affecting your gut, such as food sensitivities that cause inflammation, bacteria overgrowth, parasites, and emotional stress.

Replace: This step looks at digestive enzymes, bitters, bile, and betaine HCl which may be low and affecting your digestion; these could be highly beneficial when replenished.

Reinoculate: This involves replenishing probiotics and especially prebiotics. Taking oral probiotics is like visitors to a city. While they are there, they boost the economy. To help your microbiome population thrive, you must build your gut bacteria. Prebiotics support this process, which is crucial for long-term health.

Repair: The next step is repairing the lining of the gut, which can be achieved with soothing herbs and critical nutrients that increase the integrity of the lining.

Rebalance: Lastly, to cement all the work you have done so far and keep up the good results, we have to work on stress levels, sleeping well, and exercising. Through this Five R journey, you will know your body better. So listening to that is part of rebalancing and maintaining.

These five concepts I have learned from the Institute for Functional Medicine are life-altering when applied well to your particular needs.

Let's explore each one of the categories in more depth.

Remove

In a disease or crisis, the most obvious step is to remove what is upsetting you, aggravating you, or literally making you ill. If someone is attacking you, you can't start working on healing your wounds while the attacker is still there, picking at existing wounds and likely causing new ones.

Imagine trying to build a house. You work all day and do so well; then at night someone tears it all down, over and over again. Will you ever make progress? Probably not. Let's say you work extra, extra hard, so hard it can't all be destroyed at night. You are making some progress, but in this way, you will soon get exhausted and give up. That is how some people feel when they haven't identified this "attacker." They work hard at their health with little progress, so they want to give up.

Some of the most common assailants to remove are possible food sensitivities and allergies, infections, toxins, and stressors.

First and foremost, the removal step includes ensuring you eliminate properly every day. A good image of types of bowel movements can be seen by googling the Bristol stool chart; numbers three and four are normal.

We naturally approach the remove step when we try to eat healthier. Foods that are not serving us well create stress. Our bodies need to work harder to process inflammatory foods or those that don't provide the adequate nutrition our body needs.

The elimination diet is the first approach to remove some foods that may affect us negatively. The standard elimination diet I work with removes eight foods—or food groups, in the case of dairy. For one month, we eliminate gluten-containing foods, dairy, eggs, corn, soy, alcohol, sugar, and caffeine. Depending on where you are on your health journey, this may seem like a lot, or you may have already eliminated some of these foods.

By eliminating these foods for a month, we allow our bodies to start healing. The reactivity to those foods clears within those few weeks, and then when reintroducing these foods one at a time, we get a clearer picture if we are reacting negatively or not and identify any sensitivities.

When we do this diet plan, we see a natural shift toward more variety in your diet, typically richer in fruits and vegetables. The elimination diet is not a diet where calories are restricted, which is attractive to some people. Instead, the elimination diet plan promotes more awareness around food and our choices.

We are creatures of habit, so this is an excellent time to explore, especially with more variety in the plant world. This plan is naturally anti-inflammatory and tends to reboot the healing of your microbiome. You may notice withdrawal symptoms like headaches or low energy, but eventually, symptoms start to lessen as the gut begins to heal.

There is a particular process to eliminating these foods and their reintroduction, so I recommend you work with a healthcare provider who is knowledgeable with this type of diet.

The symptoms we may experience as a reaction to a particular food when we begin reintroducing them to our diet might not necessarily be digestive. Here are some examples of how food sensitivities may show up as symptoms in our bodies: headaches, foggy brain, sleepiness, insomnia, fatigue, nasal congestion, runny nose, depression or anxiety, muscle or joint pain, skin breakouts, itching, feeling flushed in the face, diarrhea or constipation, abdominal pain or cramping, gas, bloating, and acid reflux.

The reintroduced foods are added in their simplest form. For example, if you want to reintroduce and test for gluten sensitivity, you would have cream of wheat or plain wheat pasta. Having a pizza would not be good since it would introduce both gluten and dairy at the same time.

While the elimination diet is the gold standard, in some cases, we may be sensitive to foods that are not on that list. If GI symptoms persist or autoimmune issues are present, I recommend looking further into testing for IgG food reactions.

Food sensitivities shift depending on how often and how much you eat certain foods. As opposed to food allergies, which are generally more permanent than food sensitivities, once we heal the gut, we likely will be able to eat foods we were previously sensitive to with no side effects.

Here is the difference between allergies, sensitivities, and intolerances.

Food allergies: You have an immune system reaction, acute and fast, within minutes. Peanuts are a typical example. Allergies can be dangerous and lead to anaphylactic shock, which is an IgE response.

Food sensitivities: They are also immune system reactions; however, this is a slower and less acute response, which can happen within hours to days (IgG).

Food intolerances: Your body cannot digest food, usually because it lacks a specific enzyme. One example is lactose intolerance.

When we are sensitive or allergic to certain foods, we may crave the same food your body is reacting negatively to. This is because foods that we are sensitive or allergic to can cause an imbalance in blood sugar; in a sense, we feel the sugar high followed by the drop, and then we want that food again. Our body produces more addictive chemicals, and then we want more of that food. In addition, since we tend to eat some of the same foods regularly, we may lack in certain necessary nutrients. The body feels like it's starving, so you eat that same food again in an attempt to get more nourishment. Lastly, we may have an immune reaction, and a dormant virus may resurface, such as with a sore on the lip in the case of herpes simplex virus 1.

When trying to get a deep, peaceful sleep, the combination of inflammatory markers and blood sugar imbalance can be a real problem for some people.

Even with the healthiest foods, I like to keep some rotation schedule in mind. It doesn't have to be very strict, but be mindful of eating the same food daily. For example, most of us know coconut oil can be very healthy. However, if you eat it in every shape or form every day, a few times a day, you may develop a sensitivity. Or, a personal example, I have become sensitive to the foods I grew up with that I ate daily: gluten, dairy, and eggs.

One technique to consider and plan for your meals is the four-day rotation diet, where you tend to eat foods from the same family and then skip them for a few days, during which you focus on a different family. Or you could rotate the type of nuts, oils, protein, etc. A rotation schedule brings variety into your diet, calms sensitivities, and helps balance blood sugar.

Assessing for bacterial overgrowth, fungal overgrowth such as yeast, parasites, worms, and viruses—any offenders not kept in control in the gut—is crucial for gut healing. Working with your diet can help to mitigate these issues over time. However, with more information from a stool test, herbs, supplements, or drugs may be needed to reduce this overgrowth.

Parasites play a role in insomnia, not only due to inflammation but also because they are more active at night and produce ammonia as a byproduct. Ammonia can negatively affect the health of your neurotransmitters. Parasites can be found in various tissues in the body. Some of them are normal and even beneficial. If you struggle with insomnia and teeth grinding, this is something to look into. A stool test can give you more information on whether this is a concern, but not all parasites appear in these tests. Some practitioners like to do a parasite cleanse once a year as prevention.

The overgrowth of bacteria is often directly correlated to the levels of the beneficial bacteria found in the gut. In some people, if the beneficial bacteria are low, the treatment is mainly aimed at building the microbiome with probiotics and prebiotics, which is discussed in the reinoculate section. However, if the bacterial overgrowth is significant, a combination of antibacterial agents and building the gut bacteria compounds are used.

The removal of toxic emotional stress is equally important, as discussed in the previous chapter. Emotional stress will affect our microbiome. Studies show that stress decreases beneficial bacteria such as *Lactobacillus.* Stress is a broad term, as previously explained. In a study done in the military on the effects of stress on the microbiome, stress included psychological stress, sleep deprivation, toxins, pollutants, noise, diet, environmental pathogens, high altitude, and environmental extremes such as hot or cold, and a combination of these (Karl et al. 2018). This study showed the certain stressors have a negative impact on gut health—such as cold, high elevation and noise—while others have a positive impact, such as exercise and diet changes.

Emotional stress and trauma healing is a rather complex subject and not always easy to address. It may take time and support from a therapist, but it's all worth it. Think about it this way. If you have a strained relationship with your partner, how could you ever wholly and profoundly relax when you go to bed next to this person? Even if you put distance between you and sleep in another bedroom, which might help some, the unresolved issues remain with us. Similarly, if you have a strained relationship with yourself, it is harder to be at peace at night and let go. You are here reading this book, so you are likely trying to work on living a healthier life. It takes a personal commitment to leave the stress behind.

The sleep foundations chapter goes into more detail about this subject. The truth is, we will always have some stress in our lives. So it comes down to making a conscious decision to let go of the stress at night. Even better, work on bringing peace into your life during the day.

Replace

We ingest food every day, often with no second thoughts. We never think about this if we are blessed with no apparent digestive symptoms. However, our "digestive juices" are not as abundant as they used to be as we age. But before we explore any possible deficiencies in pancreatic enzymes, bile, or stomach acid production, let's talk about chewing first.

Chewing signals to the body that it's time to produce whatever chemicals are necessary to digest our food effectively. The ideal digestion starts with us chewing our foods enough times that they become almost liquid as we swallow. Conversely, when we drink juices or smoothies, we should chew the liquid, even though we could easily swallow it, so it mixes with our saliva and sends the signals to produce the proper enzymes.

The difference between this practice and eating your food as usual can mean extending your eating time from five to ten minutes to twenty to thirty. The first time I tried this, it felt so ridiculous. To begin with, I tried chewing each mouthful thirty times. That seemed impossible, especially with certain foods that felt like they needed almost no chewing. Then I learned that some foods may need fifteen to twenty chews while others, especially meat, need thirty or even longer.

We are told not to eat when stressed and to relax before meals. There is great value in taking a minute to say thanks before a meal or simply allowing yourself to take three deep breaths before eating. If you don't do any of that and chew as described above, relaxation will come while you eat. You can't chew that many times and not relax as chewing demands peace.

You may say, "But I don't have the time to spend so much time eating, especially for breakfast and lunch." You cannot afford *not* to take that time. Chewing will ensure that you absorb the proper nutrients. It asks us to stop, feel our bodies, and taste our food. If not, we pay later in other ways as our health declines.

When we don't chew enough, the brain gets the signal that something is off, and there is some rush because of possible danger. It can't tell that we didn't allow enough time for lunch because we need to hurry to the next meeting. It just perceives urgency, worry, and stress. Digestion is not all that important when we live in a sympathetic (fight and flight) mode. We are meant to live in that mode about 10 percent of our time—when there is real stress, a real problem. If a real problem is present, which means a genuine threat to our life, digestion of food is not all that important. After all, if I might die soon, I should use all my resources to conserve energy and be on guard, not digest food.

When we are under constant stress, real or perceived, the pancreas no longer produces healthy pancreatic enzymes to help digest carbohydrates, protein, and fat. Bile production, which further helps with fat digestion, is affected negatively. Stomach acid production can also be negatively affected by chronic stress. When the stomach acid is low, we tend to develop more gut infections, and we have a higher chance of developing bacterial overgrowth in the stomach, the small intestine (SIBO), and the colon.

If you have chewed your foods for way less than twenty to thirty times per mouthful, it can take a little practice to do better. We are not meant to swallow our foods, but that is what we are used to.

Chewing thoroughly with each meal will gradually signal the body to get into a new pattern and produce more of what we need for proper digestion.

The second way to help stimulate those digestive enzymes and stomach acid production is by taking herbal digestive bitters. The digestive bitters trigger digestion in a few different ways. Research shows that one of the most significant ways is by *postprandial hyperemia*, which is increased blood flow to the gastrointestinal system during digestion and absorption of nutrients (Kvietys 2010). The bitters are also excellent for stimulating liver function and bile production.

The third way to temporarily support digestion is by taking digestive enzymes, which will replace what your body is not yet producing. The chewing will support the production of more digestive juices; the bitters will also help and train your body to do better in time. Lastly, if you need an immediate replacement, you can take pancreatic digestive enzymes to digest carbs, protein, and fats, betaine HCl for stomach acid, to help with protein digestion, and bile acids for fat digestion at the beginning of each meal. Remember that you will return to ground zero once you stop taking them. The chewing, the bitters, and working in the relaxation response will help your body process the food properly and heal.

We can assess for deficiency of various enzymes in several ways. For pancreatic enzymes, we can test elastase in the stool. Pancreatic enzyme deficiency—exocrine pancreatic insufficiency—may cause bloating a couple of hours after eating, though not always.

The inability to properly digest fats can also show up in the stool test. When you have trouble digesting fats, you may feel nauseated and unwell when eating fats, and you may notice your stools floating in the toilet bowl.

We can usually test stomach acid insufficiency by taking one betaine HCl capsule with each protein-containing meal. If you feel discomfort or burning in the stomach area, you already produce enough stomach acid, so discontinue the use. If you take the betaine HCl capsule for a couple of days with no burning symptoms, you can increase it every three days by one capsule, up to 3,500 milligrams.

If you experience burning with a meal, you take one capsule less, which is your dosage. If you reach 3,500 milligrams and no burning, that is your dosage. It is not advised to increase the dosage any more since that is the usual amount a healthy stomach produces. One thing to pay attention to if you experience burning at any moment is to make sure your meal is average-sized and you didn't have a smaller portion, which would change your reaction.

Before trying betaine HCl, I recommend testing for *H. pylori* bacteria. Best to check stool antigen for *H pylori* not serum *H pylori* IgG as the blood test does not indicate current infection. If you have an overgrowth of this bacterium, taking betaine HCl will worsen the growth, and you may even get a stomach ulcer.

H. pylori can be treated with a round of antibiotics or with herbal medicine over two months. After testing, some patients require another two months of herbal medicine treatment to heal the infection. After treating the *H. pylori* successfully, try using for betaine HCl since one way to keep an *H. pylori* recurrence in check is having enough stomach acid.

Protein digestion is essential for sleep because if you don't break it down into amino acids, such as tryptophan, you won't make enough serotonin and melatonin.

Individuals put on acid blockers often do not have an excess of acid but just the opposite, which is unfortunate because these medications have long-term negative effects on health. Many people have a decline in stomach acid as they age, so what is more common in individuals with acid reflux is that the sphincter muscle is loose and fails to close tightly, causing food and stomach acid to back-flow into the esophagus. The more stomach acid you have, the tighter the sphincter needs to close. Another cause for acid reflux can be eating too close to bedtime, it is best to finish your dinner two to three hours before bedtime.

Lastly, healing the gut lining will improve the production of enzymes. One reason for this is the function of *cholecystokinin* (CCK). CCK is a hormone from the duodenum, the first part of the small intestine, right after the stomach, that triggers the bile and pancreatic enzymes production. If you have issues in the wall of the intestine, such as intestinal permeability issues and damaged villi, CCK production can be affected. The CCK production impairment would then affect your production of digestive juices.

The small intestine has a mesh-like barrier to only let through tiny, broken-down nutrients. If the integrity of that mesh is affected, larger food molecules can get through, and the immune system will treat these as the enemy—even if this "threat" is a large molecule from broccoli. The increased permeability may be due to poor diet, gluten sensitivity and celiac disease, high altitude exposure, or strenuous exercise. The intestines also have these finger-like projections called *villi.* Because of these projections, the square footage of the intestines is significantly increased—to a tennis court size, all to enhance the absorption of nutrients! If we had no villi, we would be seriously malnourished. Celiac disease, immune deficiencies, food allergies, food sensitivities, and certain infections such as giardia can significantly damage these villi.

Reinoculate

Reinoculating involves populating your colon with beneficial bacteria by taking probiotics and feeding your microbiome by eating or supplementing with prebiotics. Prebiotics are crucial for healthy digestion and sleep. Notice that I am talking about *pre*biotics not *pro*biotics. Probiotics are also great, but they serve as a placeholder only. While they can benefit your health, once you stop taking them, your gut will essentially be where it was before you started unless you add more and more prebiotics to your diet.

Prebiotic foods contain nondigestible fiber, which will feed and grow your beneficial bacteria. This fiber is found in some foods you may already be eating. Here are some examples: green or slightly unripe bananas, uncooked plantains, garlic, onions, asparagus, dandelion greens, endive, jicama, legumes, honey, sunchokes, and whole grains.

It takes time and consistency with these foods to improve your gut microbiome. The good news is that you can introduce these foods into your diet daily and make it seamless.

The original inoculation happens at birth, from the mom, through the vaginal canal. If you were born through a cesarean section, you have likely lived with less beneficial bacteria than those born vaginally. Having less beneficial bacteria may have contributed to your health issues, and you may need to pay more attention to prebiotics and probiotics to improve your health.

An exciting current NIH (National Institutes of Health) grant to Stanford University, along with MFM (maternal fetal medicine), is looking at the mother's and baby's microbiome. This study will investigate the diet impact on maternal microbiome during pregnancy and their infant's microbiome up to about two years postpartum (Gardner, Sonnenburg, and Karakash 2023).

The importance of maintaining healthy gut bacteria on our physical and mental well-being can be found across multiple research studies. One study has shown that a single round of antibiotics can cause depression (Lurie et al. 2015, 1522-28). Antibiotics can sometimes permanently delete beneficial strains of bacteria, most commonly *Lactobacillus*.

NSAIDS (nonsteroidal anti-inflammatory drugs) which many of us take for pain or injury support, can also affect healthy beneficial bacteria (Maseda and Ricciotti 2020, 1-20).

If we have low beneficial bacteria, the production of serotonin will likely be affected, and therefore sleep and mood will be impacted. If you lack entirely certain strains of beneficial bacteria, which you can determine through stool testing, you will need to supplement for the rest of your life with that particular strain. The prebiotics won't help with that strain since the prebiotic fiber will help grow deficient strains in your gut. If it's nonexistent, there is nothing to grow.

Probiotics are also available through eating fermented foods, though not appropriate for everyone. Some people have a hard time clearing histamines out of their bodies, so eating fermented food can have a detrimental effect. With the build-up of histamine, people have more trouble sleeping.

In addition, if you have SIBO, taking probiotics or foods high in probiotics will cause a worsening of the symptoms. We want to feed the bacteria, but since there is an overgrowth in the small intestine, the same nutrients that are meant to go to the colon will first pass through the small intestine and feed bacteria that are not meant to be there in the first place. Focusing more on diet changes and antibacterial agents in the *remove* step is more critical, followed by introducing probiotics later.

Some of the probiotic categories to consider taking, together or in a rotating manner for maintenance, are Lactobacillus and Bifidobacterium combo, *Saccharomyces boulardii*—a non-pathogenic yeast that acts as a probiotic for the prevention and/

or treatment of gastrointestinal issues (safer for SIBO), and soil-based probiotics using different bacillus species.

The saying "Eating an apple a day keeps the doctor away" can be true when it comes to gut health. The pectin in the apple accounts for 50 percent of the fiber in apples and can help increase beneficial bacteria and decrease the harmful kinds.

You can also use a blend of prebiotics in supplement form. The only caveat with prebiotics is that they indiscriminately feed all the beneficial bacteria in your gut. One of the beneficial species is *Clostridioides*. However, if it's overgrown, it can cause issues, including insomnia. *Clostridioides* will interfere with neurotransmitter balance, and sleep struggles can appear. Specific prebiotics are better than others in this case. Let's say you have overall low *Bifidobacterium* but high *Clostridioides*; you will do better by avoiding inulin types of prebiotics since they will feed both. Arabinogalactan will only support the *Bifidobacterium*, not the *Clostridioides*.

Lastly, Psyllium husk is a prebiotic powder that most people tolerate well.

Repair

Repairing the lining of the gut is as crucial as the previous steps. These "Five *R*" steps work best when taken in order. This order is not because of their relative importance, per se. They are interdependent. If only some of these aspects are addressed, the healing process may be slowed or even halted.

Intestinal permeability health is most important when it comes to sleep because of the inflammation resulting from intestinal permeability integrity issues. The intestinal walls act as a mesh. As mentioned earlier in this chapter, larger food molecules will get through when the mesh integrity is affected, and the body becomes reactive to them. Some people feel like they can only eat five foods; otherwise, they feel sick. Avoiding that many foods for the rest of your life is not sustainable so the goal is to heal the gut's integrity.

Certain nutrients will help this process. L-glutamine is an amino acid that is beneficial to heal the gut lining and reduces intestinal permeability. Shock, trauma, vigorous exercise, high altitude, chemotherapy, radiation, and significant stress reduce L-glutamine. In a study, L-glutamine supplementation shows a reduction of exercise-induced intestinal permeability issues (Zuhl et al. 2015, 85-93).

People who have been in car accidents, even if not majorly injured, tend to develop issues with intestinal permeability. Numerous patients have said they have never been the same since the accident. The brain-gut connection is noteworthy yet again. An article from the *Journal of Trauma* shows that intestinal permeability is present seventy-two to ninety-six hours after the initial injury (Faries et al. 1998, 1031-36).

Intestinal permeability issues affect the absorption of nutrients in the gut lining but also impact digestive enzyme production, as mentioned earlier. The inflammation process is more acute than if the lining was healthier, and there may be more food sensitivities and the body struggling to deal with toxins and infections. Insomnia often follows because of this.

You can add soothing herbs and nutrients, such as marshmallow root, slippery elm bark, aloe vera, and zinc carnosine.

It is always wise to start simple, especially initially, as the gut may be susceptible and even react to certain herbs or nutrients. You may start with L-glutamine for the first few weeks and then add a formula that has L-glutamine plus the herbs and nutrients listed here.

In addition, as mentioned in the online genetics chapter, if you know you have variants in the glutamate and GABA genes or notice that taking L-glutamine makes your sleep worse, it might not be the best supplement for you.

Bone broth can also help heal the gut lining mostly because of the collagen found in it. This drink can be a seamless addition to your diet.

Rebalance

The rebalance step wraps it all together. It encourages the healing process along the way and prevents relapses. Rebalancing is about learning what your body likes and sticking with it. It's also about what we do outside of nutrients and supplementation.

Sleeping well is one of the central components of the rebalancing step. This book is for the people who can't sleep. They know how vital sleep is because they lack it. To the insomniac, nothing is more triggering that we can talk about. In this section, though, I will briefly cover why sleep is essential for healing your gut and your health in general.

Sleeping well will help you rejuvenate, let go of stress, and dive deeply into complete parasympathetic mode. Research shows not sleeping well affects the gut microbiome negatively. It puts the body into fight or flight mode. Many patients report feeling nauseated, lacking appetite, and even experiencing stomach pain because of a bad night.

When we don't sleep well, beneficial bacteria decrease, the immune system function may be affected, and we have an increased chance of insulin resistance.

If you are reading this book, you are likely not consciously pushing yourself not to sleep but just the opposite. Telling you more about how sleep deprivation affects your well-being may create further anxiety. However, this may explain why healing may take a little extra time for people with insomnia. But once enough potential has been built, you will see actual and consistent results.

The rebalancing step involves a healthy amount of exercise. On that note, light and moderate exercise can be very beneficial to heal from insomnia and also for prevention. More intense exercise done earlier in the day is ideal, with lighter exercise, such as walking or yoga, later in the day, including in the evening.

Managing stress levels is another important matter. If not addressed, stress will create a negative loop, and it'll be much harder to heal. Resolving and managing stress is covered in various parts of this book. Stress relief is crucial since all the insomniac types are affected by stress, emotional and other stress.

Blood sugar imbalances

Blood sugar and sleep have a tight and close relationship and, unfortunately, can form a vicious cycle; blood sugar issues can cause insomnia while insomnia can further exacerbate a blood sugar imbalance.

The brain uses a large amount of sugar at night and relies on quick, direct energy. If there are any fluctuations at night, you will wake up since the body perceives the inability to gather quick energy as dangerous. The body sounds the alarm, as sugar is needed for vital functions. With that wake-up, there is a rush of cortisol because of its close relationship to sugar production. Cortisol is a glucocorticoid whose primary job is to raise blood sugar. Its other main function is to work with the stress response.

As you remember in the previous pages, I mentioned how this relationship between blood sugar fluctuations and sleep can cause sleepless nights. In the case of hypoglycemia, when glucose is not readily available, the body will perceive that as stressful, and you will wake up in the middle of the night feeling wide awake. On the other hand, in hyperglycemia, more cortisol will be produced, which excites the nervous system and may lead to insomnia.

Before diving deeper into blood sugar, let's look at the seasonal connection. When we are not in sync with seasonal variations in light fluctuations, we live against how we were programmed to live. Light-and-dark cycles and rhythms regulate hormone production.

The circadian rhythm runs on a twenty-four-hour cycle. For women, we have monthly cycles, such as the menstrual cycle, or even larger cycles of life, such as menarche to menopause. The seasonal cycle influences the activity of the immune system, so being in touch with the seasons is essential. We sleep more in the winter, which means more time for the immune system to replenish, deal with viruses, and adjust to the cold.

Melatonin, for example, not only has a circadian rhythm but also a seasonal one. Melatonin is produced less during the day and more at night. In addition, melatonin production is higher in fall and winter and lower in spring and summer. It also tends to be lower at hotter temperatures and higher at colder temperatures.

Regarding digestion, until the modern era, we ate according to the seasons. In the summer, the days are long, and light is plentiful; we eat more carbs, and the body knows winter will come at some point, hence a certain degree of famine. It craves more carbs to store the excess as fat to live on in the scarce season that is about to come. With artificial light, though, we live in "perpetual summer" and tend to eat more carbs typically year-round. We tend to store more fat. We then also become more insulin resistant. In addition, exercising too vigorously will also tend to raise cortisol. Now my body says not only is famine coming because it doesn't know the perpetual summer exists, but a lion is also chasing me due to strenuous exercise. T. S. Wiley discusses the Forever Summer Syndrome in his book *Lights Out: Sleep, Sugar, and Survival* (Wiley 2000, 1-6).

Chronic cortisol elevation due to stress—emotional, physical, environmental, mental, etc.—creates this perception where you constantly feel rushed. Even time perception is modified and surreal. You feel like you never have enough time to do what you need to, and you must push a little longer to finish your work. Then the body wants more energy.

Since quick energy comes from sugar, you go for it. Cortisol rises as its primary job is to increase blood sugar. Like when you are under threat and need to run, your body produces cortisol, giving you more blood sugar and fueling the body to run. But that is a problem with sleep. You may even get a bump in adrenaline, which can cause heart palpitations and even cause you to break out in a sweat. Then you are up, wide awake.

In Chinese medicine, we emphasize the need to live, eat, and sleep with the seasons. Just because everything has changed over the last hundred years since artificial light has been abundant in our households doesn't mean our bodies' biological ways have changed. *There hasn't been enough time to evolve to these new patterns.*

Living in balance with the seasons is not about returning to the old ways but using our technology to thrive. We have choices, and we can exercise them every day.

Low blood sugar is problematic for sleep issues, and so is high blood sugar. The brain needs constant glucose to function well. It relies on it and doesn't do well with converting it from fat. As previously mentioned, the body will alarm to get more sugar by increasing cortisol in the body and, therefore, waking you up.

Another side effect of low blood sugar is that it can lead to higher cell death, which produces calcium. Calcium is excitatory and will make you more likely to experience sleepless nights. Some people supplement with calcium at night, along with magnesium, and typically, that amount of calcium will not cause sleep issues. However, magnesium is calming to the nervous system, and when taken with calcium, the relaxation response is not as powerful since the two compete for absorption.

High blood sugar will cause a different kind of problem. Too much sugar in the cell will cause oxidation, specifically, advanced glycation end products (AGEs). Those AGEs damage the nerves, including the ones related to breathing, and are, therefore, a contributor to sleep apnea.

Developing insulin resistance creates a yo-yo reaction, with the blood sugar vacillating between too high and too low. When you have insulin resistance, your body will produce more insulin, which is pro-inflammatory. Inflammatory markers are perceived as stress in the body and hence another reason why sleep can be affected.

Insulin increases fat storage and also growth in the body. This insulin function can be especially problematic in women, as the insulin and higher fat storage will influence hormone levels such as estrogen, progesterone, and testosterone. Estrogen dominance, polycystic ovarian syndrome, and other hormonal imbalances arise. Insulin resistance is often associated with high triglycerides, a type of fat in the blood. High triglycerides induce leptin resistance. Leptin is a hormone made from fat cells, which helps reduce hunger. If you are leptin resistant, you will be hungry more often. Decreased leptin sensitivity has been associated with sleep fragmentation in mice (Hakim et al. 2015, 31-40).

Your doctor can check your glucose, fasting insulin, leptin, and HbA1c—your blood sugar average over the past two to three months. A calculation that can be used to detect early insulin sensitivity is the HOMA-IR calculator, which you can find online, which uses your fasting insulin and glucose; under two units shows that you are insulin sensitive. This is good. Over two units shows that you are starting to become insulin resistant, which is not so good.

You can also check your blood glucose at home by purchasing a finger stick glucometer or a continuous glucose monitor and testing your blood sugar throughout the day. The only possible issue is that these monitors are not always accurate. You can check for accuracy by coordinating a close reading to a morning blood draw.

You can test your blood glucose with a finger stick glucometer at home this way. In the morning, before eating, within thirty minutes of waking up, it should be between seventy and ninety mg/dl. Test your blood sugar two hours after breakfast and two hours after dinner; it should be under 140 mg/dl or ideally under 120 mg/dl.

A wonderful alternative for testing blood glucose, commonly used for people with diabetes, but growing in popularity as a way to improve health in nondiabetic individuals, is a CGM (continuous glucose monitor). CGMs can offer twenty-four/seven information about your blood sugar trends related to sleep, nutrition, and exercise. I have used CGMs personally to optimize my nutrition and have recommended them often to my patients. Each and every one of them have learned things about their blood sugar that improved their health, and some of them moved from the prediabetic stage to normal blood sugar levels within a couple of months because of the help of this valuable tool.

Signs that you may be experiencing blood sugar issues are:

- feeling hungry easily
- feeling hungry at night (or sometimes simply waking up at night)
- feeling lightheaded and anxious
- fatigue
- irritability
- recurrent yeast infections

More serious signs are:

- sweating
- blurry vision
- slow healing sores
- tingling and numbness in hands and feet
- swollen and bleeding gums

Note that some of the symptoms may surface about four hours after eating in what is called *reactive hypoglycemia*. Reactive hypoglycemia typically happens because of a meal high in carbohydrates and low in fat, protein, and fiber. The blood sugar will spike as a result of a high carb meal, and then once the insulin is produced in response to move the sugar from blood into the cell, the sugar in blood will drop fast and significantly and will cause the reactive hypoglycemia.

An interesting research study shows that infections with *H. pylori* causing gastritis may cause hypoglycemia (Acbay et al. 1999, 1837-1842). *H. pylori* stimulates gastrin secretion, which stimulates insulin, causing hypoglycemia. *H. pylori* can be treated successfully with specific supplements and herbs such as DGL (deglycyrrhizinated licorice), mastic gum, marshmallow root, and aloe.

Blood sugar balance depends on minerals such as vanadium, chromium, and zinc. An overabundance of toxic ("heavy") metals can interfere with the blood sugar balance. The Toxic Burden chapter dives deeper into the subject of toxic metals.

Healing blood sugar imbalances

Healing blood sugar issues involves assessing what we eat and how we eat. The food plan that heals blood sugar imbalances is high in protein, fats, and non-starchy vegetables that don't create blood sugar spikes.

I recommend small amounts of starchy vegetables to help provide quick energy and replenish glycogen levels. However, with insulin sensitivity, start with tiny amounts, like a couple of tablespoons of starchy food, or wait to introduce them until blood sugar levels are more stable.

To assess which foods are best, we must understand the glycemic index and glycemic load.

The glycemic index is a relative measurement of how quickly a food will increase your blood sugar. The scale goes from zero to one hundred, with foods with a glycemic index under fifty-five being low, fifty-five to sixty-nine being medium, and seventy and above being high.

The glycemic load is a measure that will tell us what proportion of a particular food will elevate blood sugar. It is calculated by multiplying the glycemic index by the net grams of carbohydrates in the meal. This accounts for the portion size you eat and, therefore, is a more rounded and complete way of assessing the impact on your blood sugar. Low glycemic load is one to ten, medium glycemic load is eleven to nineteen, and high glycemic load is twenty and over.

It is essential to consider both since some foods have a high glycemic index but low glycemic load; for example, watermelon has a high glycemic index, as high as a doughnut, but a much lower glycemic load than a doughnut—eight (low) for watermelon versus seventeen (medium, trending high) for a doughnut. Another example would be for half a cup of boiled carrots: the glycemic index is a whopping ninety-four, but the glycemic load is 3.9 (which means small amounts of carrots are accepted while high amounts can cause a blood sugar spike).

To work on healing the blood sugar imbalance, favor foods with both lower glycemic index and glycemic load. When eating foods with medium or high glycemic load, eat them with protein, fiber, and fat to dampen the impact on blood sugar. Ensure you digest protein properly; otherwise, the body won't get appropriate nutrition, and you will crave more carbs, which make sugar.

As a general rule, the more refined a food is, the higher the glycemic load is; the more fat and fiber a food naturally contains, the lower the glycemic load.

Limit your caffeine because it stimulates the adrenal glands, which produce cortisol and increase blood sugar, creating a negative cycle.

To fast-forward blood sugar healing, use diet changes along with a CGM, as mentioned previously, because it will provide instant feedback on what is working for you and what can be changed.

Fasting to heal blood sugar imbalances

Intermittent fasting is another choice for healing blood sugar issues as it can help balance blood sugar and improve insulin sensitivity.

Before going further, note that I generally don't recommend intermittent fasting to individuals with blood sugar issues who have insomnia. But it can be done successfully in some people.

There are several types of fasting:

Time-restricted fasting is the easiest one to do. Most people can do this type of fasting, which involves restricting their eating period to eight to twelve hours. I often advise my patients to practice a twelve-hour overnight fast, which is relatively easy for most. If you eat dinner at 7 p.m. and have breakfast at 7 a.m., you are practicing time-restricted fasting.

Some of us may naturally be doing that; others may need to skip the evening or middle of the night snack to achieve this.

Fasting intervals (or alternate day fasting) involves a one-day restriction of calories to no more than six hundred, eating as usual the following day. For some people, restricted fasting can be done every third day instead of every other day.

Intermittent day fasting reduces calories to as low as six hundred a specific day of the week. This type of fast is usually done for twenty-four hours.

Fasting mimicking diet is done five days per month. A study has shown that after three consecutive cycles of fasting for five days for three months in a row, there is improvement in markers such as fasting glucose, triglycerides, cholesterol and C-reactive protein (which becomes increased in inflammatory conditions) (Wei et al. 2017, 1-13). The ProLon Fasting Mimicking Diet is a meal program that could assist you in successfully completing this type of fasting.

Here are a few things to remember before fasting when you have sleep troubles and you are likely living on stress hormones.

If your insomnia has started due to chronic stress, and you likely have an imbalanced cortisol curve, fasting may not be the best place to start. As you go longer and longer without a meal, the blood sugar will run low, and one of your body's reactions is to produce more cortisol to help manage the blood sugar issue. Since you are already running on an imbalanced communication between the hypothalamus, pituitary, and adrenals, these spikes will prevent you from healing and possibly worsen your insomnia.

Even the overnight fast will cause problems for some people, as some will benefit from a complex carbohydrate snack to help with blood sugar and increase tryptophan levels, which increases serotonin and melatonin.

I highly recommend starting with a balanced diet of three complete meals daily as you begin healing your sleep. You may start with a twelve or thirteen-hour overnight fast to begin with and then, eventually, you may extend that time to fourteen to fifteen hours.

If you do decide to do some fasting to heal insomnia, make sure you eat a balanced breakfast (including twenty to thirty grams of protein). A protein-rich breakfast will set you up for more balanced blood sugar levels throughout the day. Women do better fasting during the *luteal phase*, the period of time between ovulation and bleeding; fasting during this period of the monthly cycle will positively influence the menstrual cycle and any PMS symptoms.

Menopausal women can benefit from a thirteen-hour daily fast as a strategy to prevent breast cancer (Marinac 2016, 1049). However, shorter periods didn't have the same effect. An example of a thirteen-hour fast would be 7 p.m. to 8 a.m.

If you decide to go with a more extended type of fast, follow the instructions below, but I recommend that people start this only after they are already sleeping better and as long as it doesn't affect sleep quality.

Drink plenty of water, add electrolytes, and keep your exercise mild to moderate. Use a CGM to monitor your blood sugar and watch for low or high blood sugar trends.

Some individuals may feel dizzy or lightheaded as they start fasting; if these symptoms persist or you have any concern at any time, talk to your provider.

If you have diabetes, metabolic syndrome, or recurring hypoglycemia, also work with an experienced practitioner. Fasting is also not recommended in pregnancy, while breast-feeding, for those with eating disorders, low BMI (body mass index) or otherwise underweight or frail, low blood pressure, and the insulin-dependent diabetic. For the safest results and to answer any questions related to your particular situation, talk to your doctor before trying fasting.

Supplementing for blood sugar healing

Diet is vital to normalize blood sugar levels. However, herbs and supplements can be helpful to speed up the healing process.

Natural alkaloids like berberine, which is healing for both the gut and blood sugar levels, bayberry, and supplements such as lipoic acid, chromium, and vanadium are beneficial in balancing blood sugar levels.

Many herbal adaptogens such as ashwagandha, holy basil, and rhodiola will help regulate blood sugar and cortisol levels.

Omega-3 fatty acids will help heal the insulin receptors and membrane health. The same with vitamin D levels; adequate levels help with healthy blood sugar levels since vitamin D receptors are in the pancreas.

Acupuncture for digestive healing

Acupuncture has been used for thousands of years in China to treat digestive disorders. While some promising research is showing its efficacy, we need more clinical research studies.

Based on present research and my clinical experience, acupuncture is helpful by increasing and regulating GI motility to improve bowel movement; it also increases gastrointestinal organ function and activity (Li et al. 2015, 8304-13).

Acupuncture can improve the gastrointestinal barrier to prevent intestinal permeability, especially in combination with moxibustion (Shang et al. 2015, 4986-96). Lastly, it modulates and improves the gut-brain axis (Fang et al. 2015, 1-11).

Step-by-step action items

- Observe your digestion and see any trends; for example, if you tend to get bloated after eating, try the betaine HCl challenge.
- Be aware if certain foods tend to make your more restless, agitated and anxious, or make your sleep worse.
- Look at the *Five Rs* and assess what may be imbalanced.
- Do an elimination diet and see how it affects your sleep and overall health.
- Make a point to try a new vegetable or fruit each time you go shopping to increase variety in your eating.
- Check your blood glucose health with blood tests and use a CGM to optimize blood sugar health.
- Work with a practitioner to further assess your digestive health.

CHAPTER TEN

HORMONES

Aim of this chapter

- Learn why hormonal health is so important to heal insomnia.
- Understand what a normal cycle is.
- Understand how insomnia can appear through the various parts of a twenty-eight-day cycle and how insomnia relates to sex hormones.
- Learn how hormones affect men's sleep.
- Continue learning about adrenal health and how it connects to sex hormones.
- Understand thyroid health as it relates to sleep.
- Have an understanding of various tests to assess hormonal imbalances.
- Understand the various factors affecting hormones, such as liver function, gut health, and blood sugar.

- Understand the next steps to start the healing process, foundational herbs, supplements, and therapies to consider for healing hormones and sleep.

Hormonal changes are one of the most common culprits for insomnia, especially for women over thirty years of age. Hormone fluctuation during reproductive years, perimenopause, menopause, and postmenopause can influence the quality of your sleep greatly.

Women struggling with hormonal changes have constituted the larger percentage of my patients throughout the years.

The hormones that will be mainly discussed in this chapter with regard to women are reproductive hormones such as estrogen, progesterone, and testosterone.

We discuss testosterone and estrogen imbalances for men because they can contribute to insomnia and sleep apnea.

However, this chapter will focus more on women's hormones since hormones influence their bodies more widely than men.

Hormonal imbalances influence a woman's health for most of her life. The hormonal shifts can be a blessing but also an immense source of pain and frustration. They are a blessing because our hormonal changes gauge our health, but these hormonal fluctuations can be debilitating for some women. Having suffered from terrible menstrual periods, I understand this. If years of pain weren't enough, perimenopause kicks in for some of my patients with a new set of issues. If insomnia wasn't present until then, this is a prime moment for it to surface. Unfortunate timing since sleeping can support this transition process greatly.

Supporting your hormones is a lifetime of commitment. I wish there was some magic bullet, but it truly is about tending to your hormone health every month. The more I heal and watch other women heal, the more I see working on hormonal health as an effective way to attend to your overall health. The body always gives you signs when something is not quite right, and the menstrual cycle and all that comes attached to it is a significant way through which we gain valuable hints.

The trouble is, though, most of us are not doctors or healthcare providers. The education we receive in school about our bodies is so minimal it could be considered worthless. Worse, great shame is attached to our bodies, especially our menstrual cycles. We explore more of how your body works in this chapter followed by practical ways to help you feel more empowered and in charge of your body.

It is important to look at hormonal health and how it impacts your insomnia. Hormonal insufficiency, such as low progesterone, can cause sleep issues. Adequate progesterone levels are essential for sleep because sufficient progesterone increases GABA activity. GABA will make you feel relaxed. When deficient in GABA, you tend to ruminate, overthink, and be more anxious.

Estrogen dominance, either high due to *xenoestrogens* (chemicals that act like estrogen) or simply high estrogen compared to progesterone, can affect sleep quality.

Hormonal changes cause temperature fluctuations, hot flashes, and/or night sweats. This temperature change is especially true at perimenopause and menopause. Our temperature is meant to be steady and low at night; any fluctuations will pull you right out of sleep. Hormonal changes are among the most common reasons women have sleep disturbances. Low hormones can also lead to muscle loss and increase the chance of sleep apnea.

High testosterone, which is common in PCOS (polycystic ovarian syndrome), often affects the circadian rhythm and may cause insomnia, especially trouble falling asleep. HPA (hypothalamic-pituitary-adrenal) axis dysfunction may be more apparent during perimenopause and menopause. With unbalanced cortisol levels and low DHEA (dehydroepiandrosterone), the adrenals won't produce enough steroid hormones, and that small amount of hormones is crucial when the ovaries quit producing sex hormones. Low testosterone in men and women can be a contributor to insomnia.

Thyroid function will affect the quality of your sleep; it may cause either hypersomnia or insomnia.

Learning to track your menstrual cycle by taking your temperature every day of the month and keeping a score of your ovulation will prepare you when subtle changes happen before symptoms are severe. Understanding the types of insomnia you develop because of menstrual cycle changes will help you feel more empowered and knowledgeable when you talk to your provider.

Assessing to see if you have hormonal issues

Women's hormones

Hormonal imbalances can be subtle or obvious. What is crucial to establish, regardless of one's struggle with sleep, is what a normal cycle is. For example, this culture tells us that painful cycles and clots with each menstruation are normal. But is that true?

While everyone is different, we see certain common characteristics with a healthy menstrual cycle. Your cycle should be between twenty-five and thirty-three days. For some women, it can be a little longer or shorter and still be considered normal but not very typical. What is essential is that it is consistent for you.

Menstruation bleeding typically ranges from three to seven days. The flow should be manageable, usually not changing your pad/tampon more than three to four times in twenty-four hours, not too light with barely any flow, or with no extended spotting. A heavy flow is losing over eighty milliliters of blood or using more than eight super pads in your entire period. An average loss of blood is around thirty-five to forty milliliters.

A healthy color for your menstrual blood is darker red; brown, pale red, and bright red can all indicate specific dysfunctional patterns in functional and Chinese medicine.

No clots should be present in your blood; in Chinese medicine, clots represent "stagnation." Clots could be due to stress, an unhealthy diet, or your liver's inability to process your hormones effectively. They can also be due to fibroids and endometriosis.

The second part of the cycle, the *luteal phase* consisting of ovulation day through the next bleeding cycle, is at least ten days long, ideally twelve to fourteen. A short luteal phase may cause fertility issues and indicate deficient progesterone among other things. It could also cause you to feel irritable before your cycle with preperiod spotting, breast tenderness, and insomnia.

It is normal to feel slightly less energetic during your

bleeding period and a few days after. However, being in pain, suffering from headaches, and being very tired is a sign that your hormones are not as balanced as they could be. In healthy cycles, we feel most energetic, interested in sexual activity, and alive around our ovulation.

Breast tenderness, irritability, sugar cravings, and insomnia the week before your bleeding are abnormal and show a possible imbalance in estrogen and progesterone.

Ovulation should happen every month, or mostly every month, if you are in your reproductive years. Ovulation is a sign that the normal hormonal fluctuations within your body are abundant and healthy. Ovulation can be observed by watching the cervical mucus change to egg-white consistency and taking your basal body temperature.

Transition into perimenopause and menopause can be smooth; you don't have to suffer endlessly through night sweats, hot flashes, and insomnia. Feeling a particular change in your body and mind is normal. However, it should not completely turn your life upside down.

A year or two after menarche, around sixteen years old, I started having intense, heavy, and painful periods. These lasted through my teens, twenties, and now in my thirties; it's still not "perfect." Because I have been in the health field for over fifteen years, the less-than-ideal menstrual cycle has constantly reminded me to work on my hormones.

Remember, we are not striving for some perfect ideal for our monthly cycles but reaching for a place where we notice we get healthier and healthier. A place where we understand our bodies and don't feel out of control and lost when we experience symptoms. Insomnia especially is a big symptom to understand since it usually leads to anxiety, fatigue, and simply being incapable of leading a normal, happy life.

Insomnia and hormonal fluctuations

Insomnia can show up some typical ways due to hormonal fluctuations.

- You may have trouble falling asleep or wake up in the middle of the night during the second part of your cycle, especially the week before you start bleeding. You may have increased night sweats and/or hot flashes during the same period, one week or so before bleeding. Less commonly, some women wake up early in the morning around 3, 4, or 5 a.m., the few days before bleeding.
- Again, not as common, but you can also experience insomnia right around ovulation for a day or two. One "smart" reason for this may be because this is optimal time for conception, and it is normal for a woman to be more aroused or interested in sexual activity at this time in her cycle.
- You may have trouble sleeping when you start bleeding or a couple of days in. More intense dreams may show up the few days before or during your menstrual bleeding time.
- Skipping periods but still having PMS symptoms without bleeding can also happen. One of my patients calls these "phantom periods," all the "fun" symptoms such as irritability, insomnia, and bloating but not actual bleeding.

Trouble sleeping, in general, may not be connected with the cycle itself but may have developed due to heavy bleeding causing low iron. Many of my patients are not yet clinically anemic, but they are borderline and have insomnia either as described above or throughout the month to varying degrees.

Insomnia can be worse with stress. The connection between possibly imbalanced hormones, cortisol, and blood sugar cravings can create the perfect storm for sleepless nights.

To properly look into hormonal imbalances, we must look past the sex hormones produced in the ovaries. We step back and see what else is closely connected to these hormones. The thyroid influences virtually every organ in the body, including the reproductive organs and hormones.

The adrenal glands regulate the stress response, among other things, and greatly influence how the thyroid reacts. The next section will discuss the proper order to heal your hormones. The order makes all the difference regarding the success of your healing journey.

Thyroid health

Thyroid health is crucial since some sex hormone issues are due to impaired thyroid function. Thyroid hormones, particularly T3, affect LH (luteinizing hormone), which stimulates the ovaries and testicles and therefore affects estrogen and testosterone levels.

Low thyroid function can increase the risk of having cystic ovaries and affects ovarian health in general.

This being said hyperthyroidism (an overactive thyroid) can show up with sleep issues.

Some of the common symptoms of hyperthyroidism are:

- irritability
- feeling hot
- losing weight
- palpitations

- tremors
- increased sweating
- increased bowel movements

What I see more often than hyperthyroidism is the autoimmune disorder Hashimoto's. Since Hashimoto's is autoimmune hypothyroidism, it typically leads to increased sleepiness.

However, the picture can be a little more complicated than this. This autoimmune hypothyroid condition can show up with temporary swings into hyperthyroidism. This swing happens because as the demand for thyroid hormones increases since it's in a hypo state, the thyroid can temporarily swing into a hyper state and lead to temporary insomnia.

Another fact to consider is that when the thyroid is imbalanced, there are likely adrenal and sex hormone imbalances. So even though theoretically we should be able to sleep a lot, though many times we're still tired even after nine or ten hours, many of my patients experience insomnia.

Another consideration to remember with Hashimoto's disease, is that it is an *autoimmune* disorder. One of the prerequisites to developing Hashimoto's disease is a gut imbalance along with a genetic predisposition and a trigger—remember, most of the immune system is located here. As explained in the previous chapter, gut imbalances can also be at the root of your sleep issues.

Some of the most common signs and symptoms of hypothyroidism (low function):

- fatigue
- *hypersomnia* (needing to sleep too much)—though insomnia is often present

- weight gain
- dry skin
- brittle nails
- hair loss
- constipation
- memory lapses
- menstrual issues
- increased sensitivity to cold

Adrenal up-regulation due to stress will affect thyroid hormone conversion. In these cases, the TSH (thyroid stimulating hormone) will show up as normal while the levels of the active form of thyroid hormone T3 may not be ideal, which can lead to typical hypothyroid symptoms.

To get a complete reading of your thyroid function, these are the blood test markers: TSH, free T4, free T3, reverse T3, and thyroid antibodies. In autoimmune thyroiditis, a small percentage won't even have elevated thyroid antibodies, which would indicate autoimmune activity; an ultrasound is then advised if autoimmunity is still suspected to see if there are any changes to the thyroid gland.

Reproductive hormone health, stress, and sleep

Before diving into sex hormones, addressing adrenal health along with thyroid health is essential. We addressed adrenal health and the stress response in the previous chapters.

The basic idea is that imbalanced cortisol will influence the production of estrogen, progesterone, and testosterone as well as their ability to bind to receptors.

In the following paragraphs, I will present two main scenarios on how stress affects reproductive hormones. The first one, the "pregnenolone steal," is where I start when I consider hormone imbalance in my patients. The second scenario is HPA and the sympathetic adrenal (SA) axis uncoupling, which we already discussed in the stress response chapter. We are focusing more on the first scenario because it relates directly to reproductive hormone health.

The stress response causes a generalized priority pyramid. Procreation is not a priority when in chronic stress; hence the reproductive hormone levels are affected during stress.

The steroid pathway has given me a nightmare or two because it is so complex. But if you stay with me here, I think I can help you understand how it's all connected.

Reproductive hormones start from cholesterol—hint, not all cholesterol is terrible—which will make pregnenolone. From there, the pathway splits in two. One branch makes DHEA (dehydroepiandrosterone), which in turn will make estrogen and testosterone. The other branch will produce progesterone, which will make cortisol.

When chronically stressed, cortisol can take too much from the progesterone pool. The cortisol steals too much energy from pregnenolone, where the progesterone comes from; that is called a "pregnenolone steal." If this goes on long enough, it will deplete the pregnenolone even more, and then the other pathway, which goes into DHEA and in turn makes estrogen and testosterone, also gets depleted. Now progesterone is deficient, which will appear as estrogen dominance. But again, if this goes on long enough, even estrogen will become deficient, along with testosterone.

The pregnenolone steal is a debated theory, and by some accounts, the HPA axis is affected instead, as explained in the stress response chapter. The medical community is not always in agreement with the concept of the pregnenolone steal because they say that the primary source of energy, the mitochondria, which are the powerhouses of cells, don't share their pools of resources in that way, where the body can "steal" from another area.

However, there is undoubtedly an imbalance in cortisol, and it may instead be due to what we call the *sympathetic adrenal (SA) axis uncoupling*, where the cortisol and adrenaline systems separate and don't seem to communicate. We thoroughly covered the adrenal imbalance in the stress chapter. No matter what the processes are, exactly, managing stress to heal your hormones is crucial for insomnia.

Testing women's hormones

Types of tests to look into with a health care provider are the urine hormonal tests such as the DUTCH Plus (Dried Urine Test for Comprehensive Hormones); it not only gives in-depth information about hormones but also their metabolites and which pathways your body favors to eliminate them.

This in-depth information is crucial to know, for example, because estrogen can prefer certain pathways more prone to growth including cancer. This test includes saliva tubes to test cortisol levels. Saliva sex hormone tests will give similar information though without the breakdown of those essential metabolites.

Both the saliva and urine tests will also give your cortisol and DHEA levels. Blood is necessary to assess SHBG (sex hormone-binding globulin) levels.

Hormonal testing to assess progesterone and estrogen levels are done on day nineteen through twenty-one for menstruating women—to be more exact, five to seven days after ovulation.

Men's hormones

Hormone imbalances in men can cause insomnia, especially testosterone deficiency and estrogen excess. In particular, testosterone deficiency has a close relationship with sleep. Lack of this hormone will cause more insomnia and can be associated with sleep apnea while not sleeping will diminish testosterone levels.

Unfortunately, *hypogonadism,* characterized by low testosterone, is surprisingly common in the US. An epidemiological study showed that 38.9 percent of men forty-five and older had low testosterone (Mulligan et al. 2006, 762-769).

Addressing potential thyroid issues is vital because thyroid hormones, in particular T3, affect LH, which stimulates the testicles and therefore affects testosterone levels.

Unfortunately, we see more and more younger men experiencing less than optimal testosterone levels, affecting many aspects of their lives.

Low testosterone levels may cause symptoms such as: low libido, infertility, erectile dysfunction, fatigue, muscle fatigue, longer recovery after exercise, insomnia, depression, sleep apnea, weaker bones, osteoporosis, and thinning hair as you get older.

High estrogen comes with its own set of issues, with similar symptoms as low testosterone, and often can happen simultaneously. Estrogen will cause weight gain, and the fat itself will further increase the amount of estrogen, increasing risk of stroke and heart attack—since there is an increased risk of clotting—and of prostate cancer.

To understand how to balance these hormones and improve sleep, we must first address why these hormones go haywire. Stress is a significant factor in increasing the activity of some of the enzymes that dysregulate hormones; aromatase will increase the estradiol conversion from testosterone while 5-alpha-reductase will increase the conversion from testosterone to DHT (dihydrotestosterone). The 17,20 lyase enzyme, found in fat, brain, and skin, will stimulate testosterone conversion to estrogen. All these conversions lead in one way or another to low testosterone and/or high estrogen. Some men take medications to inhibit 5-alpha-reductase to shrink an enlarged prostate—treatment for BPH, benign prostatic hypertrophy—or to prevent hair loss.

High estrogen can cause hot flashes, insomnia, erectile dysfunction, infertility, and gynecomastia, which is enlargement of breast tissue in men. Xenoestrogens from personal care products, plastics, etc., increase estrogens and lead to estrogen dominance.

Low testosterone—also favoring the DHT pathway I mentioned above—can cause sleep issues, fatigue, low sex drive, hair loss, loss of muscle mass, and even increased body fat and poor memory.

Insulin resistance affects the balance of these hormones, along with excess weight.

High SHBG (sex hormone binding globulin) will bind bioavailable testosterone, which leads to lower levels of available testosterone.

Taking statins (cholesterol-lowering drugs) may decrease testosterone since cholesterol is the building block of testosterone.

High cadmium can lower testosterone levels. High cadmium levels are found in present or previous cigarette smokers and well and possibly tap water; read more in the toxic burden chapter.

Testing for reproductive men's hormones

Men with health issues such as erectile dysfunction, low libido, depression, fatigue, or loss of muscle mass should have their total and free testosterone, SHBG, cortisol and thyroid hormone levels checked.

The thyroid and adrenal glands must work optimally to successfully heal from sex hormone imbalances. Assess thyroid health by blood testing for TSH, free T4 and T3, reverse T3, and thyroid antibodies. Autoimmune thyroiditis is much less common than in women.

Prostate health should also be assessed through a combination of blood testing and physical exam if indicated.

The DUTCH (Dried Urine Test for Comprehensive Hormones) test will give you a comprehensive view of hormones, including the 5-alpha-reductase, aromatase enzyme activity, and cortisol.

Lastly, you may assess for LH and SHBG levels in the blood.

It is essential to understand and see the levels of the mtabolites before doing replacement therapy because in individuals who have insulin resistance, alcohol issues, too much stress, and who are obese (or overweight) and inflamed, the activity of both aromatase and 5-alpha-reductase leads to elevated estrogen and DHT (dihydrotestosterone). The DUTCH test measures these metabolites, so working with a practitioner familiar with this testing will be beneficial.

Vitamin D

Vitamin D (ergocalciferol) is actually a hormone, not a vitamin. It has receptors in the brain and is essential for sleep. Vitamin D is needed for gut and immune health as well as to produce acetylcholine, which is necessary for good rest (Watson et al. 2010, 513-528).

Vitamin D is increased by exposure to the sun. Sunlight is the driving force for healthy circadian rhythms, so I recommend everyone to get outside within the first hour after waking up or use a light therapy lamp when getting outside is not ideal.

Some people have genetic variants such that daily exposure to the sun is never enough to achieve optimal vitamin D levels, so checking vitamin D levels in the blood—more specifically, 25-hydroxy vitamin D—is recommended in both the summer and winter to assess what is normal for you and whether supplementation is recommended or not. While the conventional laboratory normal range is thirty to one hundred ng/mL, optimal levels of vitamin D are between sixty and eighty ng/mL.

Heal your hormones and improve sleep

Healing women's hormones

Healing your hormones is crucial for sleep support. There is no way around it, and it's a large part of our body's functioning from puberty until the moment we die—less so after menopause but still crucial for many women.

We celebrate taking a birth control pill so we don't have to deal with a cycle. I don't blame you; who wants to be in pain, bleeding profusely, or suffering from migraines each month?

Nobody. But our hormones and the rest of the body work through a feedback mechanism for a reason. As attractive as it is to take a pill to override this mechanism, we have to think of the long-term effects it has on our bodies.

As we dive into the healing process, let's consider a few things about our hormones.

Progesterone peaks in the third week of the menstrual cycle. When progesterone is sufficient, we sleep better, feel happier and more relaxed, and have slower bowel movement transit times, smartly designed to have time to extract more nutrients in case of pregnancy.

Progesterone lightly diminishes insulin sensitivity, and it can therefore increase blood sugar imbalances. We all know the feeling of being "hangry"; this would be an excellent time to focus on eating adequate amounts of protein to avoid overeating sugar, which increases inflammation and leads to more painful periods. We are designed beautifully, though; with the increased appetite in this period of time, our bodies smartly ask for extra nourishment just in case of possible pregnancy.

Estrogen is the caring and loving hormone, but it's too stimulating to the nervous system when high. The fourth week of the cycle can be an issue with sleep. This higher level of estrogen can be due to a true deficiency of progesterone, or it can be because of a ratio problem where the estrogen is too high in comparison to progesterone. Xenoestrogens can be a causative factor, from environmental sources such as plastics, cosmetics, etc.

If there is an estrogen deficiency or a significant drop before menstruating, it will lead to lower serotonin, which will also cause more sugar cravings and feelings of depression.

Not ovulating means no *corpus luteum* release, which produces progesterone during the second part of your cycle.

Progesterone tends to dominate the second part of the cycle, which is why unbalanced estrogen dominance is a problem. Progesterone is soothing to the nervous system, and likely the week after ovulation may be your best time of the month for sleep.

With hormone levels declining as you approach your period, you are more likely to have trouble sleeping. Also migraines and headaches may kick in.

Some women experience insomnia at ovulation because, for a short period of time, the hormones are low following ovulation. Another sign that the levels of hormones right around ovulation have dropped too much is spotting, which happens right before progesterone rises to more adequate levels. Always check with your doctor if you have irregular bleeding or spotting.

Managing stress and exercising, especially after ovulation, is crucial. High cortisol will block the progesterone receptors and hence cause more insomnia. This response is yet again an intelligent design of the beautiful bodies we have: if we are stressed, the body will say, "It's not a safe time for entering pregnancy; responding to the big bad danger is wiser right now" (the body cannot differentiate if it's just that you are stressed about a deadline or that a tiger is constantly trying to get you).

Research shows a connection between melatonin production and progesterone levels, with melatonin possibly stimulating the progesterone (Caufriez et al. 2011, E614-E623). This is particularly important since melatonin levels decrease as we age, which may worsen women's symptoms during perimenopause and menopause.

Understanding your body through taking your basal body temperature

Taking your basal body temperature is an easy, affordable way of getting to know your body and your cycle better. These types of thermometers connect with an app on your phone and can help for either birth control or conceiving. They are not 100 percent accurate by themselves as a birth control tool, but when combined with checking for changes in vaginal fluid, this method can be more precise.

Your temperature will climb half a degree to one degree at ovulation time and stay up until you bleed again. On day one of our cycles, we start bleeding, which lasts a few days. The temperature stays pretty stable until the day after ovulating, around day fifteen for most women.

The temperature fluctuations tell us that LH has surged, and you likely have ovulated. With that surge, the estrogen and progesterone levels start increasing. As this happens, the temperature will stay higher until progesterone drops significantly after ten to fourteen days, once the endometrium is ready to shed, if you are not pregnant. The moment the temperature drops, you start bleeding within hours.

Taking your basal body temperature will inform us of a few things. It can hint whether you ovulate. When you ovulate, the body releases the egg from the corpus luteum. The corpus luteum produces most of the progesterone in the second part of the cycle. Progesterone is thermogenic, accounting for the temperature rise.

It can also tell us the length of the second part of the cycle, the luteal phase, which is crucial since having a short luteal phase could hint at low progesterone, vital to conceive and maintain a pregnancy, and very important for your sleep.

When approaching perimenopause, when we take our temperature, we feel more empowered as we can notice skipped ovulation or a change in our cycles and be more prepared for the transition before any other symptoms arise.

Knowledge is power. As we get to know our bodies, we understand our lows and highs, our sexual desires or lack of them, our moods, and the times when we can likely get pregnant and when we cannot.

These basal body thermometers connect to an app on your phone and cost thirty to fifty dollars. After a few months of tracking, you start seeing a pattern and learning more about your body's rhythm. More complex devices can cost around two hundred dollars, and some of them can test LH and estrogen. The more detailed devices are most valuable if you are trying to conceive.

It is essential to take your temperature around the same time, within thirty minutes to an hour, in the morning. As soon as you wake up, check your temperature before getting out of bed since standing up will slightly raise the temperature. Once you do it for a while, this becomes a habit. If you have had a bad night of insomnia, the temperature may not be as accurate.

Accuracy is best when you have had at least four hours of consecutive sleep, ideally in the last part of the night. Keep this in mind but don't worry too much about it. Just take your temperature every morning; after a couple of months, you should be able to see a trend.

For urine hormone testing, you generally collect samples on day nineteen through twenty-one of the cycle. Since only some women ovulate on day fourteen of their cycles, it is more important to keep in mind testing five to seven days after ovulation rather than day nineteen through twenty-one of the cycle.

I ovulate each month on day seventeen. Years ago, before taking my basal body temperature and knowing exactly when I ovulated, I collected the saliva sample on day nineteen, thinking that would be good since it's five days after day fourteen. The results came back showing my hormones were low. But the reality is, based on my ovulation time, I collected the sample only two days after ovulation instead of five to seven days. There was not enough time for the healthy spike of hormones to happen. A few months later, I collected the sample on day twenty-three, which showed healthy hormone levels.

Some women can tell exactly when they ovulate because of mild discomfort in the ovarian area. If you haven't yet kept track of your cycle with basal body temperature, you can purchase LH strips to determine your accurate ovulation day. When we start working together, I recommend this to my patients to make sure the hormone test we are about to do is collected at the perfect time of the month.

However, the LH spike can sometimes be missed, even when measuring, since it can be present in urine metabolites for just a few hours. For example, if the spike happens in the afternoon and you always test in the morning, you can miss it. If you use the LH strips, start testing once daily with your first-morning urine around day seven of your cycle. Day one is the first day of bleeding.

As you approach the expected ovulation, I recommend testing the LH twice daily. Some more advanced ovulation devices test both LH and estrogen and can be even more accurate than just using the LH strips.

Being aware of your hormonal fluctuations throughout the month is incredibly empowering. I would like to share this section on taking your basal body temperature with all the women in the world. I would start by teaching our teens and young women about their menstrual cycles. After all, to a certain degree, our menstrual cycle shapes many decades of our lives.

GALS and hormonal health

As a general rule, we are looking at four aspects when it comes to hormones:

1. how to produce higher amounts of hormones
2. how to better transport hormones in the body
3. how to work on hormone sensitivity receptors
4. how to support the detoxification of hormones

To make these processes as efficient as possible, I use the mnemonic GALS from functional medicine. I learned this during my training at the Institute for Functional Medicine:

Gut—The gut is in constant communication with your hormones through the receptors found in its lining. If you have constipation, IBS (irritable bowel syndrome), or inflammation in the gut, it will affect the hormones, especially estrogen.

Adrenals—The adrenal glands send bursts of cortisol when in need, usually due to stress, to help you manage the situation. But when this happens chronically, it starts to affect the health of your hormones.

Liver—The liver helps process and detox hormones; factors such as a toxic environment, alcohol consumption, and genetics can all overwhelm the liver and lead to hormonal imbalances.

Sensitivity and Sugar—receptor sensitivity is crucial for sex hormone health. The response that the body receives from these receptors up-regulates or down-regulates the amount of usable hormones in the body. Sugar metabolism and insulin resistance will affect hormone levels as well.

The gut and women's hormones

This section discusses how the gut affects hormones, especially estrogen. However, since the ratio of estrogen to progesterone is critical, this section is of prime importance for issues related to progesterone deficiency since estrogen can become dominant in this scenario.

Hormones are produced in the ovaries. Once in circulation, they are processed with the help of the gallbladder and liver. They then enter the gut to be eliminated through the stool. Some of the estrogen gets reabsorbed—a small amount of metabolites is optimal—but most of it is excreted.

The particular part of the microbiome that helps with estrogen metabolism is called the *estrobolome*. The estrobolome refers to the bacteria in the gut that help detox and break down estrogen. If that detox process is affected, we reabsorb more significant amounts of estrogen into the body. Larger estrogen amounts circulating in the body promote growth and may lead to various types of cancer, fibroids and ovarian cysts, breast lumps, infertility, thyroid nodules, and endometriosis. Sleep issues can also surface with estrogen dominance.

IBS (irritable bowel syndrome) is correlated with estrogen metabolism and has been strongly associated with the gut-brain axis. Estrogens, especially sudden changes, seem to influence the microbiota and the intensity of IBS. The concept of *microgenderome* is the sex hormone modulation of the microbiota. Indeed, nothing exists and functions independently in the body; everything is interrelated.

Estrobolome health is based on healthy bacteria thriving in the gut. When certain bacteria are overgrown, they activate an enzyme called *beta-glucuronidase*, which can be tested in the stool. This enzyme reroutes estrogen from the bowels to be reabsorbed into the body in larger amounts. We want levels of this enzyme not to be too high but not too low, either. If a stool test shows low beta-glucuronidase, it signifies low estrogen. As mentioned above, it can lead to estrogen dominance and unwanted growth if it's too high.

Beta-glucuronidase feeds on *Clostridioides* species, *E. coli*, and *Bacteroides*. Though these are common species in the microbiome, when populations get too high, it's problematic. Overgrowth of *Clostridioides* species also interferes with neurotransmitter conversion, which can further add to sleep issues.

In the case of an overgrowth of these species, taking a broad-spectrum antibacterial formula can help establish a new balance in the gut. In addition, certain probiotics can be of particular help. For the *Clostridioides* overgrowth, *L. Reuteri* and *Saccharomyces boulardii* can help get the population to healthier levels.

High beta-glucuronidase can be treated by working on the microbiome. In addition, taking Calcium D-glucarate will lower beta-glucuronidase, and the gut excretes excess estrogens. Raw carrots have an indigestible type of fiber that can help bind excess estrogens. So, in this case, one carrot a day can keep the doctor away! Also, chew the carrot well or grate it. You can eat it as a snack, in a salad, or a smoothie.

To optimize the function of the estrobolome, working on the gut, as discussed in the previous chapter, is essential. For example, having regular bowel movements will help with estrogen metabolism. That is because slow transit time will allow more time for estrogen to get reabsorbed into the body's circulation.

The adrenals and hormones

We are not meant to live in high-stress mode for most of our lives. Running to appointments, clenching our teeth while writing an email, holding our breath while thinking of a conversation—it's not sustainable. When we run on this stress mode, it comes at a great expense.

The "pregnenolone steal," explained earlier, is one way we possibly get robbed of our beloved progesterone. Some people don't think this pregnenolone steal is how it happens but rather through a feedback mechanism through the pituitary, which lowers sex hormones such as progesterone. Regardless of the cause, there is a clear correlation in my clinical practice between improving stress management in a woman's life and watching her hormone levels regulate.

When discussing adrenal health and sex hormones, we must examine the HPA (hypothalamic-pituitary-adrenal) axis. You may have read about "adrenal fatigue," but the truth is the problem is not with the adrenals necessarily but more so with the body's resilience when dealing with chronic stress.

The stress response chapters along with the sleep foundation sections in this book offer many ways to slow down and find relief from chronic stress.

Herbal adaptogens that can help with the stress response are covered in the stress chapter. Some of the most commonly used are ashwagandha, holy basil, and rhodiola.

The liver and the hormones

The liver is one of the most important organs in the human body. In Chinese medicine, we call the liver "the general." And no kidding—it commands and supervises so much.

In Chinese medicine, most PMS symptoms are explained as a stagnation in the liver. Whatever the type of stressors and toxins present thousands of years ago, they understood back then that the liver was indeed connected with hormonal changes and imbalances. Many of my patients who experience worsening of their sleep issues the week before their bleeding starts have a liver imbalance. After all, everything that enters the body has to go through the liver, to be processed, detoxified, or guided where it next belongs.

When it comes to hormones, the liver does the following things: converts estrogen and progesterone, creates proteins to carry the hormones in the body, processes and eliminates hormones, makes bile, breaks down fat, and stops fat-soluble toxins. It is also intimately involved in the clotting cascade.

Toxin processing takes priority in the liver over hormones since they may be more threatening to the body's ecosystem. If your liver and the gut are busy clearing these toxins out of the body, hormone conversions come in second place. Drinking alcohol every night is an example of making the liver's number-one priority breaking down and clearing a toxin (the alcohol). Hormone processing is put on hold and comes in second. What is worse, alcohol can have an estrogenic effect on the body.

Detoxification of estrogen is done in the liver in three stages:

Phase 1 is detoxification via hydroxylation to 2-, 4-, and 16-OH. Urine testing will tell us the clearance ratio through these pathways, which ones your body favors since some are better than others, and whether you have estrogen deficiency or dominance. The DUTCH test is one of the tests that looks at these pathways.

Phase 2 is detoxification via methylation and COMT. You can read more about this in the genetics chapter, also tested in the DUTCH test.

Phase 3 is detoxification via transporter through the bile and kidneys and elimination in the colon.

Understanding these three phases will help your healthcare practitioner design a treatment plan to balance hormones and aid you in sleeping better. Testing for these metabolites will also give us a better idea of how to work on breast cancer prevention as there are ways to influence and guide estrogen to clear through better pathways.

The sex hormone binding globulin (SHBG) is a carrier protein produced in the liver for estrogen and testosterone. SHBG picks up hormones and drops them off at receptor sites where the body can use them.

The hormones come from cholesterol, so they are fat-soluble. Since water and fat don't mix, estrogen and testosterone need this SHBG carrier to transport to these receptor sites where they can get into the blood circulation and be usable for the body.

Levels of SHBG can be too low or too high. If SHBG is too low, that means too much free estrogen is circulating in the body, which we know can have adverse effects, including sleep issues.

If you have too much SHBG in your body and too many carriers, you don't have enough usable and circulating estrogen and testosterone. With low estrogen, you will often experience hot flashes, night sweats, and insomnia.

An overburdened liver will affect the production of this carrier protein and the levels of your hormones. This carrier protein can be increased by various factors, such as the liver struggling with its function, the use of oral birth control, smoking, and stress.

Low thyroid function is associated with low SHBG, and therefore, more estrogens circulate in the body and increase body weight. Then the fat itself will produce even more estrogens.

To increase SHBG, thereby decreasing usable estrogen, focus on a more vegetarian diet, eat one to two teaspoons of flaxseed per day, supplement with green tea catechins, correct possible vitamin A and C deficiencies, treat hypothyroidism if present, and treat obesity.

To decrease SHBG, thereby increase available estrogen, focus on exercising, especially resistance training, use omega-3 fatty acids, optimize vitamin D, assess testosterone levels, work on insulin resistance, and heal metabolic syndrome.

Insulin receptor sensitivity and hormonal health

Insulin is like a key that takes glucose out of the blood and unlocks the gate to allow it to enter the cell. We want the cells to be very responsive to insulin. If the receptors are resistant, we need more insulin, which activates inflammatory gene pathways. High insulin increases fat storage and also tends to boost growth.

For women, insulin resistance has been linked to estrogen dominance. For some women, insulin resistance can cause high testosterone, which can cause PCOS (polycystic ovarian syndrome). Women with PCOS will have trouble falling asleep or self-proclaim as night owls when, in fact, they tend to produce melatonin later at night due to hormonal imbalance and insulin resistance.

The body becomes more sensitive to insulin during sleep, so if a pathology surfaces, this will be more apparent at night. Sleep-deprived people have a decrease in insulin sensitivity, which makes it harder to handle glucose and tends to increase cravings.

Women are most insulin-sensitive in the morning; hence women should eat breakfast. If you're a woman considering fasting, you can find better strategies than skipping breakfast, as opposed to men, who can do better with fasting in the morning. Research shows that a high-protein, larger breakfast with an average lunch and a light dinner can diminish cravings, help weight loss, and improve insulin sensitivity (University of Missouri-Columbia 2011).

As noted in the GI chapter, various types of fasting improve insulin receptor sensitivity. Two important things to remember when designing your fasting are favoring breakfast; and, if choosing the five days fasting per month, do this after ovulation, since fasting before may impair ovulation. In addition, fasting after ovulating will likely improve your PMS symptoms.

Low blood sugar imbalances and PMS symptoms have some similarities; in both situations, you may feel moody, irritable, headachy, dizzy, anxious, and so on. Progesterone is higher in the luteal phase and tends to decrease insulin sensitivity. So if you already have some blood sugar issues, they will be highlighted around this part of your cycle.

By eating high-quality protein and fats while staying active and avoiding sugar and alcohol, you will feel better every month and sleep better.

The thyroid

The thyroid is one of the most vital organs in our bodies. It communicates with many different organs and it has a lot to say. Communication between the thyroid and sex organs goes both ways; however, when it comes to treatment, it is essential to check for thyroid function and adrenals before directly treating the sex hormones.

To work on thyroid healing, we must understand what affects thyroid function. Nutrients that help the production of thyroid hormones are iron, iodine, zinc, selenium, vitamin E, B2, B3, B6, C, D, and tyrosine. Most of these can be tested through a micronutrient panel.

Infections, certain medications, radiation, fluoride—which is an antagonist to iodine—food sensitivities, pesticides, heavy metals, chemicals that are hormone disruptors, and stress all affect thyroid function.

Since most thyroid issues are autoimmune based, especially in women, it is vital to heal the gut and determine what triggers may have started this entire autoimmune attack. For my thyroid, it was a combination of a genetic predisposition combined with gluten sensitivity, which led to more food sensitivities, high *H. pylori* infection, a *Blastocystis hominis* parasite infection, and a root canal infection that, in time, spread into my jawbone. None of these made me very sick to the outside viewer; however, my thyroid antibodies were approaching one thousand, when normal is under thirty-five, which meant my immune system was gradually attacking my thyroid.

Thyroid medication can aggravate already deficient estrogen by activating the breakdown of estrogen and making insomnia worse.

Thyroid function is complex, so if you suffer from thyroid issues, I recommend Dr. Izabella Wentz's book on Hashimoto's disease, *Hashimoto's Thyroiditis: Lifestyle Interventions for Finding and Treating the Root Cause.* She has personally struggled and healed from thyroid issues, and out of that came an incredible book that has helped so many with thyroid dysfunction.

For the perimenopausal, menopausal, and postmenopausal women

Perimenopause is one of the most common periods in a woman's life when she may develop insomnia. Perimenopause—literally meaning "around" menopause—is the period of time when hormone levels start shifting, and their production by the ovaries starts to decrease. Perimenopause can be as long as fifteen years but a general average of seven.

You can expect to feel your body changing. However, it is not "normal" to suffer throughout this period, just like we are told it's "normal" to have painful periods. Perimenopause is also called the "menopause transition." Menopause is the time when a woman's periods stop. Menopause is official after at least one year without a period.

After a woman has not bled for over a year, the following stage is the postmenopausal period. However, we commonly refer to it as being in menopause instead of postmenopause.

Many sleep disruptions happen because of the many reasons already presented in this chapter. But since this is one of the largest pools of women who experience insomnia, here is another summary from the point of view of perimenopause, menopause, and postmenopause.

Progesterone starts declining before estrogen does, which more easily creates estrogen dominance. The declining progesterone can affect sleep quality since progesterone is soothing and calming and helps GABA production. When progesterone drops too early in the luteal phase, the estrogen is too high in comparison, and we experience more irritability, breast tenderness, and insomnia the week before the bleeding period. As we start skipping ovulation, there is no corpus luteum to produce progesterone, which can worsen insomnia for some months.

With the gradual estrogen decline, hot flashes and night sweats appear, making sleep hard, with frequent awakenings, especially around 1 or 2 a.m. With estrogen in decline, we have less of an inclination and patience to be taking care of everyone, being the caregiver, etc. If levels drop too low, we may hit extreme emotional swings. As one of my patients said, she became "a bitch on wheels." Kidding aside, while this is an opportunity for transformation, which is good, change can come without feeling intense emotional distress on top of relentless insomnia.

As the ovaries reduce their production, the adrenal glands secrete a large enough amount of hormones to keep you healthy, happy, and sleeping; however, if you have functioned on high stress over the years, the production of these hormones will not be as smooth, and your body will struggle more, including with worse sleep.

As the estrogen decreases, there is a certain amount of bone loss; when this happens, minerals such as calcium get transferred from bone to blood. Heavy metals stored in the bone for years or decades also get released from bone to blood. Those heavy metals are now circulating and can harm your health and sleep. Testing and treating high levels of heavy metals is essential, ideally before this transition period of menopause—more on heavy metals in the toxic burden chapter.

If you are reading this book and are already in the middle of this period, work with a practitioner to assess whether heavy metal toxicity may affect your health negatively.

If you are not yet there, the absolute best gift you can give to your thirty-something or forty-year-old self is to take care of your hormones gradually. We tend to believe that nothing can touch us in our twenties, but usually, as we enter our thirties, especially if motherhood is part of that period, it is time to tend to our bodies and hormones.

Healing herbs and supplements for women

Healing our hormone imbalances involves a step-by-step approach based on the root cause. Some direct hormone support that can be used while finding out the why are the following:

- Maca is an adaptogen; however, the phenotype (color), dosage, and quality are all important; the phenotype will highlight whether it is better for fertility, perimenopause, or menopause.
- Vitex (chaste berry) is a wonderful herb, best used in tincture form, that can increase progesterone, balance LH, and affect prolactin levels; it's best to take during the second half of the cycle.
- Evening primrose oil may help regulate progesterone and estrogen levels, and it is anti-inflammatory as it lowers prostaglandins. High prostaglandins often lead to painful periods.
- Black cohosh can help with estrogen imbalance, especially for perimenopausal and menopausal women with hot flashes and night sweats.
- Wild yam extract can be helpful for menopausal symptoms because of its progesterone support.

Try seed cycling, though remember that the seeds need to be freshly ground and some people may react negatively to them because of food sensitivities. Seed cycling works by taking one tablespoon of raw ground pumpkin seed and/or ground flaxseeds from day one of your period until the day you ovulate. Then, take one tablespoon of raw ground sunflower and/or sesame seeds from the ovulation day through the first day of your period. The first part supports healthy estrogen production and the second part progesterone production.

A similar idea applies to oils. Fish oil can be used for the first part of the month, and borage or evening primrose oils for the second part of the month.

Chinese herbs are prescribed based on individual needs as far as dosages and combinations of herbs go; herbs are never given alone and, when combined, work synergistically.

Detox supplements such as DIM (diindolylmethane) for Phase 1 liver detox can be beneficial and help estrogens steer away from the most dangerous pathway (4-OH). DIM comes from cruciferous vegetables. Eating broccoli or broccoli sprouts is healthy, but DIM supplements deliver more quickly. Note that having symptoms of estrogen dominance does not mean we can benefit from DIM automatically. Some women will have both low estrogen and progesterone, though estrogen is still higher than it should be compared to progesterone. DIM is not recommended in that case, so it's essential to test.

Sulforaphane is also found in cruciferous vegetables and can help all three phases of estrogen liver detox. Here is a partial list of cruciferous veggies: arugula, broccoli, broccoli sprouts, bok choy, Brussel sprouts, cabbage, cauliflower, collard greens, kale, mustard seeds and leaves, radish, and rutabaga.

Foods in the carrot family (*Apiaceae*) help reduce the 4-OH estrogen metabolite as part of the Phase 1 liver detox. Some of the foods in this family include carrots, celery, cumin, anise, parsley, and fennel.

You can remove alcohol, sugar, and caffeine from your diet and see sure improvement. If you rely on those drinks and foods, it might be challenging to make this change, but I promise it's worth it.

Assessing DHEA levels and appropriate supplementation can improve your hormone imbalance.

Many other supplements will help to improve hormonal health and sleep. Work with a practitioner to identify what is appropriate for you.

Healing hormonal imbalances in men

As a man, healing your hormones is essential for your overall health and healing insomnia as well as sleep apnea, if present. Working on adrenal and stress response health is vital, as presented in the stress response chapter. Next, support your thyroid health by assuring you have all the necessary nutrients, as mentioned in the previous pages, while working on any infections, endocrine disruptors, and food sensitivities.

If you have testosterone deficiency, find out why. Do not automatically settle for getting hormone replacement. If you are overweight or obese, work with a practitioner to help you lose weight, as it affects the health of your hormones and, consequently, your sleep.

If you are on statin drugs, work with a practitioner to find possible alternatives because lowering your cholesterol may lower your testosterone.

Choose HIIT (high-intensity interval training) types of exercise instead of cardio and endurance, which tend to lower testosterone.

If DHT (dihydrotestosterone) is high, work on inhibiting 5-alpha-reductase with nutrients and herbals such as saw palmetto, quercetin, omega-3 fish oil, green tea, flaxseed, zinc, chrysin, turmeric, pumpkin seeds, and beta-sitosterols, and check on adequate progesterone levels.

If estrogen is high due to accelerated aromatase, look into the possible causes of it, such as excess alcohol, zinc deficiency, central (abdominal) obesity, insulin resistance, leptin resistance, inflammation, stress, and imbalanced cortisol.

Use aromatase inhibitors such as flaxseed, resveratrol, dietary fiber, green tea, quercetin, chrysin, and zinc. Avoid endocrine disruptors, as listed by the Endocrine Society, such as pesticides, biocides, plastics, food contact materials, cosmetics, and others (Endocrine Society 2018). Researching the products you are using will help you assess if those products or materials are safe to use. Eating organic food will reduce your exposure to some of these endocrine disruptors.

Address SHBG (sex hormone binding globulin) levels, if elevated, by taking herbs and nutrients such as stinging nettle, omega-3 fatty acids, and sufficient, high-quality protein.

When it comes to testosterone production, make sure that cadmium is not elevated; oral chelation with EDTA (ethylenediaminetetraacetic acid) can help reduce cadmium in the body while selenium helps ameliorate toxic cadmium levels until they are brought down.

To increase the general production of testosterone, replenish vitamins A and D, and use herbs such as ashwagandha, which helps with the stress response, too, and *Mucuna pruriens.*

Improve prostate health with botanicals such as rye grass pollen extract, red maca, and nutrients such as zinc, vitamin A, and selenized yeast.

Eat multicolored food, healthy fats, adequate high-quality protein, and plenty of cruciferous vegetables.

A note of caution, only take supplements with arginine if you know you don't have genetic mutations in the nitric oxide genes; l-arginine can build in the body if you cannot convert it and cause more inflammation. Arginine can also trigger HSV (Herpes simplex virus) outbreaks.

Last but not least, always work on your daily stress management.

Vitamin D optimization

You can replenish your vitamin D levels by going out in the sun; however, that may not be enough for people with genetic variants predisposed to deficiency. Furthermore we have to be aware of the risk of skin cancer with excessive sun exposure. Direct supplementation with vitamin D is then recommended. It can also be obtained from beef liver or cod liver oil.

The general recommendation for sun exposure is twenty minutes per day. Some general guidelines recommend that for levels below 60 ng/ml, add 1000 IU of vitamin daily for every ten units under. So if someone is at thirty, take three thousand; always retest to check levels.

Acupuncture for hormonal healing

Acupuncture treatments for hormones are one of the most noninvasive effective treatments I have experienced. The flexibility of adjusting needles based on which part of the cycle you are in, plus the use of Chinese herbs, makes the treatment so effective.

These treatments can regular hormonal health and improve sleep for both men and women.

Step-by-step action items for women

- Start tracking your menstrual cycle by taking your basal body temperature and logging it in the app along with the dates of your periods.
- Take notes in the same app related to your sleep, and see if there is a correlation with the time of the month.
- Eliminate sugar, alcohol, and caffeine, and notice any differences in your body or do an entire elimination diet as presented in the GI chapter.
- Clean up your pantry, laundry, bathroom, bedroom, and any other space where there might be endocrine-disrupting chemicals. Check the toxic burden chapter for additional information.
- Test your sex, adrenal, and thyroid hormones with a practitioner so you can get a better idea of what is happening in your body; choose a more holistic practitioner who will order a more in-depth test for sex and adrenal hormones, such as the DUTCH test.
- Work on digestion and blood sugar balance to support hormonal health.
- Work on stress relief.
- Receive acupuncture treatments.

Step-by-step action items for men

- Test your sex, adrenal, and thyroid hormones with a practitioner to get an idea of your levels. Choose a more holistic practitioner who will order a more in-depth test for sex and adrenal hormones, such as the DUTCH test.
- If you are taking statin drugs, pay particular attention to the relationship between cholesterol and sex hormones and work with a practitioner who understands this connection.
- Work on stress relief.
- Receive acupuncture treatments.

CHAPTER ELEVEN

TOXIC BURDEN

Aim of this chapter

- Understand how our toxic environment and our exposure to it can affect sleep
- Why toxins matter when it comes to sleeping well
- Identify sources of toxicity in your environment
- Know the various types of toxins that may be influencing sleep negatively
- Provide testing resources
- Learn the best steps to start a detoxification process

When we think of toxic exposure regarding sleep, we may first think of whatever is in our bedroom, perhaps what we sleep on. Indeed, mattresses can be filled with an unsettling amount of chemicals that are off-gassing for months.

We spend one-third of our lives in bed and in a most vulnerable situation, too—sleeping. When we sleep, our defenses are lowered more so than during the day.

The exposure to toxins and how they affect our health is much broader than what comes from our mattresses. It's in the foods we eat, the air we breathe, and the personal products we use.

We are regularly exposed to small amounts of toxins such as pesticides; because of the small amounts of exposure, we are sometimes told not to be concerned. But the small amounts matter, as many of these chemicals interact with our hormones, and our hormones interact with our gene expression. Those small, or large, amounts of each chemical not only interact with our hormones, but the chemicals themselves interact with each other.

We likely don't understand the consequences of this highly chemicalized world. While the Environmental Protection Agency lists forty-nine thousand chemicals, the number of chemicals found in circulation is twenty-five thousand to eighty-four thousand (Environmental Protection Agency 2023a; Institute of Medicine of the National Academies 2014, 5-24). This is a massive number of chemicals, very few of which have been tested, and barely any on how they interact or their consequences.

These toxins affect your body in many ways, regardless of how, exactly, they create stress in the body. We have been exposed to various toxins for as long as humanity has been around. It is conceivable that our bodies can deal with a certain amount of toxins. But when the scale is tilted incorrectly, when the input is larger than the output and/or the detoxification pathways are overwhelmed, we experience illness.

Toxicity becomes a problem when there are just enough toxins and susceptibility toward certain issues in our body that these chemicals can overpower our capability to heal. The vulnerability could be a genetic predisposition or the liver being overwhelmed already because of other problems, such as clearing alcohol out of our bodies.

In short, we are what we drink, eat, breathe, touch, and cannot eliminate. The moment we come in contact with something, whether in the form of food, the makeup we apply, or a container we eat or drink from, it impacts our bodies.

There are two types of toxins, *exogenous* and *endogenous.*

Exogenous toxins are the ones that come from the outside environment.

Endogenous toxins are the byproducts of certain compounds in the body.

A good example is mold. Mold is an exogenous toxin; however, once in the body, it produces its byproducts, affecting our health, especially when we can't eliminate the mold properly. We'll discuss mold more in the next chapter. Many of these byproducts are inflammatory and stressful and tend to increase cortisol and other stress hormones.

The toxic impact on our bodies is three-layered:

- Are we able to eliminate the exogenous toxins?
- How do the toxins interact with our hormones, GI tract, nervous system, and other systems in the body?
- Lastly, how do these toxins affect our immune system, and what consequence does that have?

Pondering these questions will reveal how sleep can be affected by toxins. As you have noticed in the other chapters, everything is truly interconnected, even though we have some defined categories like hormones, GI, etc. The relationships and interactions are as important as figuring out the root cause.

With chronic disease, the pathological changes become like a domino effect, one piece affecting the other. As much as we would like to heal insomnia by fixing it piece by piece or going backward layer by layer, the way to healing is forward and accepting that it's not about feeling like you used to feel but finding a new you.

Assessing your toxic burden to see if it's affecting your sleep

We have gotten so used to our world that we don't even notice how we may be exposed to chemicals at every step. You may wake up on a traditional mattress with toxic fire-retardant chemicals, covered with treated wrinkle-free sheets, likely made of synthetic materials.

Let's continue and see what else may happen during an average day. You leave your bed filled with fire-retardant chemicals and synthetic wrinkle-free sheets. You go to the bathroom and probably use soap, lotion, and makeup laden with artificial fragrances and endocrine-disrupting chemicals. You may use an antiperspirant with aluminum and lipstick with lead in it.

You head to the kitchen, and because you are in a hurry, you use the microwave to heat your milk and cereal, which likely contains artificial sweeteners and coloring, along with hormones in the milk that was fed to the cows. You sit on the front porch to enjoy the fresh morning air, but you're probably inhaling harmful herbicides from your treated lawn or your neighbor's lawn.

Next, you get in your car to head to work. You sense the "car smell," but you're used to it and don't realize how you are inhaling chemicals and touching the steering wheel with chemicals absorbed through your skin every day. You get to work and pass a coworker with a pleasant smell, yet again inhaling more chemicals from the artificial perfume.

I could go on, but I will stop here. I bet you get the message. I don't want to scare you but rather to help you open your eyes and identify what you can do to lighten the body's chemical burden so you can heal.

Many things in our environment could be affecting our sleep—not just in the bedroom, but all over the house, in the yard, in the car, and in the office. We love wrinkle-free sheets, fresh-smelling pillowcases, dry-cleaned clothes, and many other conveniences. They are nice, and regrettably over time, they're damaging to our health.

Possible chemical and toxin exposures may surround us, but since this is about sleep, we'll concentrate on the bedroom.

Before we dive into this chapter and find the sources we may be exposed to, it is worth noting that many of us have been desensitized to all the smells around us.

People with multiple chemical sensitivities and environmental illnesses can be affected by conditions other people consider normal. For example, before I knew about chemical sensitivities, I realized that hanging out around a scented candle led to headaches. Or that sitting in a car with an air freshener also didn't feel good. Millions and millions of people use these products without a clear understanding of how they may affect their health. Of course, plenty of toxic elements are odorless but equally harmful.

Bedroom exposure

According to the Environmental Protection Agency, some pollutants are three to five times higher indoors than outdoors (2023b). This fact may sound surprising, but if you think about it, whatever you use is now contained in an enclosed space. The primary exposure when we sleep in our bed comes from mattresses, along with pillows, sheets, furniture, paint, candles, and flooring (Oz et al. 2019, 9171-9180).

Many of the things we use in the bedroom give off VOCs (volatile organic compounds) and are petroleum-based. It's essential to pay attention to VOC exposure since you may spend eight hours breathing them in while you sleep with your face and nose pressed close to the mattress and linens. Regarding the sources of VOCs, they can come from various places. Examples of such exposures are fragrances, petroleum-based compounds, and natural woods such as pine and natural essential oils. So VOCs are not all bad. However, sensitive individuals may not react well, even to the natural ones.

Some of the fibers we use in our bedrooms may have been treated with herbicides and fungicides. What is meant as a protective measure—making products fire retardant—comes back to damage your health in other ways. The convenience of our lives, such as having wrinkle-free materials, also can come with a price tag attached. The process of making wrinkle-free sheets commonly includes using the chemical formaldehyde.

Learning about what lives in your bedroom is very important, so you can make better decisions and ensure these chemicals don't cause or add to your sleep problem.

One of the significant problems with the number of chemicals in our households is that they often overwhelm our livers. The liver has over one hundred functions in the body. One of the major functions is helping us detox. If the liver is overburdened by the chemicals in your house, it will do a poor job. For example, women experience hormonal imbalances because the liver can't correctly transform and convert those hormones.

So we attempt to identify what we are exposing ourselves to and do our best to remove those exposures—from toxins in your bedroom and household items to heavy metals from food.

Pollen, dust, and pet dander may also increase your body's inflammation and aggravate your sleep issues. They can cause nasal congestion, often seen in patients with insomnia, and sleep apnea.

Note that, for some of you, reading the next few pages may feel overwhelming because of the many changes needed to clean up the environment. However, know that you can start making changes gradually to manage the time and financial commitment that may be required.

Your mattress

Commercial mattresses are, unfortunately, a source of exposure to more chemicals than you ever imagined—a combination of chemical retardants, polyurethane compounds that emit VOCs, and PVC or vinyl covers.

Many of these are endocrine disruptors and can affect your health negatively, potentially your sleep. At the very least, if these chemicals stress your body at night, your fight-or-flight chemicals will kick in, and your sleep quality will decrease.

Your linens

I grew up on a farm with no washer or dryer. The clean smell of sheets came from the outside air. If you ever had the opportunity to sleep in air-fresh clean sheets, you know how soothing that is. No wonder we tried to invent chemicals that mimic that smell. The "smell of clean" should be odorless unless you hang your linens outside, not the scent of perfumes that come from detergents. I keep my detergent as chemical-free and odorless as possible. If I want a hint of lavender on my pillow, I spritz a mixture of water and lavender essential oil.

First, the sheets, pillows, and blankets can give off VOCs because many fibers are petroleum-based. The cotton, unless it's organic, is often grown with herbicides and pesticides. Thankfully, blankets and linens can be washed in hot water, and most of these chemicals are likely washed away. The problem, then, is more with the detergent we use repeatedly.

The detergents we use may have a cocktail of chemicals: artificial fragrances, surfactants, fabric brighteners, and EDTA (ethylenediaminetetraacetic acid). The synthetic fragrance world is a deep well with unknown issues. A "fragrance" can be made out of literally hundreds of chemicals with few regulations around the term. Most of these chemicals are known to be skin irritants. We don't fully understand how these chemicals may influence your sleep, but we know they can be endocrine disruptors. The endocrine system regulates hormones, reproduction, mood, and sleep.

Some of these toxins are also carcinogenic. Whether it will affect us enough to see fundamental negative changes coming up as a disease depends on the quantities that accumulate in our body, our ability to cope, and our genetics.

The last major part of laundering your sheets is fabric softeners. They add yet another combination of chemicals. Fabric softeners are unfortunately linked to triggering asthma, skin issues and some impurities found in them may be linked to cancer (Geller 2022). Thankfully, some alternatives, such as wool balls, do not cause any side effects. Wool balls are natural, commercially available, and you can add your favorite essential oils to them. They are also an affordable investment as opposed to continuously purchasing dryer sheets.

Spot cleaners and bleach are two more products to be aware of. Spot cleaners are highly toxic, and we can usually tell by the strong smell we are greeted with when using them. Bleach can be an endocrine disruptor, affecting the thyroid gland in particular.

The effects of these chemicals may be evident in some cases, but most are subtle, and we cannot tell if they cause sleep issues. We can safely assume they may be contributing to at least a certain degree, so best to figure out the cleanest materials and safest laundering products.

Your bedroom furniture

The furniture, like our nightstands and chest, can have problems, particularly when new. Solid wood is better than pressed wood. Pine is the exception to the rule since some people are more sensitive to its VOC-emitting resins, which may cause lung issues, including asthma.

Pressed wood is made out of various compounds and glues that can be harmful. Also, water-based solvents are generally safer than oil-based solvents.

I recently purchased a new headboard for my bed, a nice velvety material. Years ago, when I knew less about these matters, I would have just said, "It's the new kind of smell; how nice." Now I wondered what I was breathing from it. So I made a point to open the window more often in the first few weeks and leave an air purifier on in the bedroom. I also let the headboard air out before installing it.

Carpet

The ideal bedroom flooring is solid wood with low natural VOCs, if you have allergies, with cleaner glues such as solvent and VOC-free adhesives.

Watch what you use for cleaning products. Avoid all waxes and chemical-laden cleaners, and always opt for natural cleaning agents.

Laminate is not ideal because the adhesive contained in the top layer emits harsh chemicals such as formaldehyde.

Carpets are primarily made from petroleum-based compounds, various sealants, and adhesives. The loom oil in new carpets is very high in VOCs because of the oils used to lubricate the machines used to make the carpets. These carpets can emit VOCs for months. When it comes to carpet padding, ask for wool padding or recycled cotton fabric.

A couple of years ago, I ran a chemical urine panel to see what I had been exposed to. I was shocked and amazed that some chemicals were five times their highest safe limit. I am healthy, always doing my best not to be around chemicals. Despite that, these test results showed otherwise. I then thought of all the new carpets I had been exposed to, the new cars, the fresh paint. They could have been what increased my body's toxicity level.

Your paint

Low- or no-VOC paints are best for the same reasons presented above. Fresh paint is worse to sleep in. According to the Department of Environmental Protection in Montgomery County, Maryland, ventilating your room for seventy-two hours is the primary recommendation (Department of Environmental Protection 2023). However, lower volumes of VOCs can emit for more extended periods of time. Make sure to ventilate properly and use an air purifier.

Your closet, dresser, and laundry room

Whatever you use for your clothes in your closet will seep into your bedroom. That may be dry cleaning chemicals, detergents, or fabric softener. It may also include mothballs, which emit toxic fumes into your bedroom.

Your nightstand

You may have scented candles and electronics on your nightstand. The scented candles often contain fragrances that may be endocrine disruptors. You may use unscented ones, candles scented with essential oils, or even beeswax-based candles which have a natural scent.

I don't know if you think of electronics as a toxin. However, EMFs (electromagnetic fields) are an outside influence that may affect your health and sleep. EMFs may be more harmful to people with a genetic mutation in the CACNA1C (calcium channel) gene mentioned in the online genetics chapter.

The subject of EMFs is highly debated, but the way I think about it is this: If the frequencies we are exposed to at night do not match the natural frequencies of the earth that we have been living on for a long time, it could affect our brains negatively.

For this reason, I recommend putting your cell phone on your nightstand only if in airplane mode and not plugged in. I also recommend not using a plug-in clock radio but prefer a battery clock instead. This way, you could even put your cell phone in another room to charge.

Earthing mats or sheets may be helpful for sleep, though walking barefoot outside on the grass every day is one of the best ways to reconnect with the earth's natural frequencies.

Various chemicals that may be affecting your sleep

Covering the various chemicals affecting your sleep can overwhelm you and me. It is rather complicated to identify and quantify which ones truly affect our sleep and to what degree.

So below, I focus on the ones I have researched and found to be either directly or indirectly related, such as endocrine disruptors or those causing inflammation.

VOCs

As previously discussed, volatile organic compounds can be found in many items, though the most concerning source is your mattress. Other sources of exposure are paints, adhesives, carpets, vinyl flooring, upholstery, air fresheners, cleaning products, cosmetics, gasoline, cigarette smoking, and dry cleaning (Minnesota Department of Health 2022).

The VOCs from your mattress come from polyurethane, and elevated heat from your body increases the VOC emissions (Oz 2019, 9171-9180). Some call sleeping with a polyurethane mattress "sleeping with the enemy."

Phthalates

Phthalate is advertised under the following names: DiNP, DiDP, DMP, DEP, and DBP. It is present in cosmetics, plastics, especially soft plastics, and aerosols such as scented candles. It is also found in some medication coating and new cars as part of the "new car" smell.

This chemical is a known endocrine disruptor, particularly affecting males. It can be associated with insomnia and leg cramps at night (Shiue 2016, 3108-3116).

BPA (Bisphenol-A)

BPA is a chemical used to harden plastics. It can be found in food and beverage packaging as well as toys. It is also commonly used in store sales receipts. Think about how many sales receipts you touch, especially if you are a cashier! Trader Joe's is one of the first stores with BPA-free sales receipts.

BPA is an endocrine disruptor that affects various metabolic processes; BPA levels are higher in individuals with severe obstructive sleep apnea than in moderate sleep apnea (Beydoun 2016, 467-476). BPA exposure has also been associated with shorter sleep.

Combustion pollutants

Nitric Dioxide (NO2), PM2.5 particles, and other combustion pollutants can harm your health. PM2.5 particles are small enough to be inhaled in your lungs and enter your bloodstream. PM2.5 particles are present in car exhaust pollution, power plants, commercial cooking, construction equipment, and industrial activities.

According to the American Thoracic Society, they have been found to decrease sleep quality (American Thoracic Society 2017). A study published by the same society has also found a link between ambient air pollution and sleep apnea (Billings et al. 2018, 1-8).

Pesticide and herbicide exposure

Pesticides may be found in many of the foods we eat every day, especially nonorganic foods. According to the EWG, some foods with the highest levels of pesticides in 2023 are strawberries, spinach, kale, peaches, pears, nectarines, apples, and grapes. Check each year for the updated "Dirty Dozen" list (Environmental Working Group 2023b).

Herbicides are used to kill weeds. The most popular herbicide is glyphosate (Roundup). According to US Right to Know, 9.4 million tons have been sprayed worldwide. To give you a better picture, this quantity is enough to spray nearly half a pound of Roundup on every cultivated acre of land in the world (Malkan 2023).

The US Environmental Protection Agency (EPA) and the International Agency for Research on Cancer (IARC) have opposing views on glyphosate health effects, the first considering it not likely a carcinogen with the latter as a possible carcinogen (Benbrook 2019, 1-16).

Bayer, the owner of Roundup, has recently paid billions of dollars to solve ninety-five thousand cancer claims with thirty thousand left to resolve (Chappell 2020).

Potential glyphosate risks are liver and kidney damage, endocrine disruption, which can negatively affect sleep, and it has been implicated in diseases such as non-Hodgkin's lymphoma.

It also has been associated with gluten intolerance, thyroid disease, infertility, and possible depletion of micronutrients such as zinc, copper, and manganese. Glyphosate may also increase glutamate, which we know is an excitatory neurotransmitter (Myers et al. 2016. 1-13; Samsel and Seneff 2013, 159-184; Cattani et al. 2014, 34-45).

Pesticide exposure, primarily occupational, has been found to be a potential risk in REM sleep behavioral disorder (Postuma et al 2012, 428-434).

Another study showed that farmers are particularly affected by pesticides, and adverse effects on sleep were observed, such as trouble falling asleep, short sleep duration, and decreased sleep quality (Li 2019, 1-11).

Low levels of organophosphates have been found to have neurobehavioral effects and cause sleeplessness, among other symptoms (London et al 2012, 887-896).

Strychnine is a pesticide that is a GABA antagonist, meaning it reduces the availability of GABA in the brain, which affects the GI and causes body stiffness and rigidity (Braestrup and Nielsen 2003, 681-684).

Organic solvents

Organic solvents are found in cleaning and degreasing materials, gasoline, paint removers, paint varnishes, adhesives, ink and ink removers, pesticides, and toiletries, especially nail polish removers. Organic solvents occupational exposure might cause sleep apnea and other sleep difficulties (Edling and Ulfberg 1993, 276-79).

Fluoride

Fluoride is found naturally in small amounts in water, soil, and foods. It has also been added to water supplies, toothpaste, and mouthwashes to prevent cavities. However, this has been recognized as a double-edged sword, and the practice has been rejected in most European countries due to its side effects (Unde, Patil and Dastoor 2018, 121-127).

Among these side effects, fluoride, along with calcium, attaches to the pineal gland; this calcification decreases melatonin production. In a study, fluoride has been shown to specifically affect teenagers' sleep cycle regulation and behavior (Malin et al. 2019, 106).

Heavy metals

Heavy metals can come from insecticides, herbicides, fungicides, dental amalgams, fish, food, supplement contamination, older homes or buildings, cigarette smoke, and air pollution.

Arsenic is found in many foods, such as shellfish and rice, and in certain countries in water as well. Along with other heavy metals, phthalates, and pesticides, arsenic has been found to negatively affect sleep and cause leg cramps (Shiue 2017, 3108-3116).

Mercury is most commonly found in dental amalgams (fillings), fish, with the highest in shellfish and large fish such as tuna, vaccines containing Thimerosal, mercury thermometers, and fluorescent light bulbs. Mercury has been associated with insomnia (Rossini et. al 2000, 32-38).

Lead can be found in paint from houses built before 1978. It has also been found in soil, pottery, some toys produced abroad, some cosmetics, Mexican candy containing tamarind, at the firing range from exposure to lead bullets, occupational exposure in auto repair, mining, and battery manufacturing. Lead has been associated with sleep disturbances, headaches, and depression (Mayo Clinic Staff 2022).

Cadmium can affect the sleep-wake cycle (Aristakesian, Kiiashchenko and Oganesian 1996, 402-408). This toxic element can damage the kidneys, so the kidneys require proper elimination and extra care for healing. Cadmium is found in present or previous cigarette smokers and water, especially well water.

Assessing for exposure

To assess your exposure to these various types of toxins, do the following things:

- Do a thorough inventory of your bedroom, bathroom, kitchen, entire house, car, office, and wherever you spend time. Write everything down that may contribute to your toxicity exposures. Read all the labels.
- Do a urine test to check for environmental toxins such as the one from Great Plains Laboratory. The GPL-Tox profile looks at 178 different environmental pollutants. This test does not include heavy metals.
- Blood tests show only acute exposure to heavy metals. However, laboratory companies such as Quicksilver Scientific Lab offer a combination of blood, hair, and urine metal analysis. The test also looks at how your kidneys and liver deal with detox.
- Another choice for testing is the "provoked urine test" or "challenge test." In this test, a practitioner prescribes a chelating agent to a person before collecting their urine to test for metals. This makes the blood test results more accurate. However, some people can have temporary worsened symptoms during and after the "challenge test." Discuss this concern with the provider prescribing this test.
- Hair tests alone can be used to assess heavy metals.
- A simple test that may show toxin burden is GGT (Gamma-Glutamyl Transferase), which is easily included in your blood panels. GGT is an enzyme in the liver that indicates a higher toxic burden when elevated.

Heal and detox so you can heal your sleep

When faced with toxins, the body has one goal—to survive—so it will do whatever it takes. The normal physiologic process is to make chemical compounds and toxins less harmful and excrete them out of the body. In this chapter, we are looking at how to maximize this natural process called *metabolic detoxification.*

There are specific steps to the detox process. Remove the source of the toxin, or at least reduce the exposure. Remember that detoxing is a complex process, and people can feel worse as they go through it if the pacing is too fast. So keep that in mind when choosing herbs or supplements, and find a professional to support you through this healing journey.

Cleaning up your environment

First, I understand that making these changes involves a financial investment. Do what you can afford and make small changes over time with purchases and decisions that are impactful.

The first step toward relieving your body from being bombarded with chemicals that may affect your sleep is to look around and eliminate what potentially could be adding to your toxic load. There is no way around these chemicals. We are all exposed to a certain amount of toxins. The healing process is more of eliminating some of what is already in our bodies and building robust elimination processes.

Start with your mattress; if it's an old one and time to get a new one, this is the perfect time to invest in one that is comfortable for your body and free of chemicals. Look for certifications such as the Global Organic Textile Standard (GOTS) and Global Organic Latex Standard (GOLS), which are considered the leading certifications for organic mattress materials, according to the Sleep Foundation (Foley 2023). If you have a mattress purchased more recently, research what is in your mattress and whether it is vital to invest in a new one.

Check that your pillows meet the same standard for GOTS and GOLS. Use sheets made of organic, natural fibers, such as cotton. Not only are you avoiding being exposed to chemicals, but natural fibers are more breathable and less likely to sweat at night.

Clean up your nightstand; make it clutter-free and phone-free. If you keep your phone on your nightstand, ensure it's not charging and on airplane mode. Keep your nightstand and your entire room clear of dust and free of artificial scented candles. Keep your closet closed, avoid keeping clothes in your bedroom that have been dry cleaned, and use natural laundry soap.

Whether you have old carpet, new carpet, old flooring, or new flooring, keep it clean and use an air purifier to clear your room of allergens, pet dander, and pollen. Wood flooring is the preferred option, if possible. Pets add more dust and pet dander; if you have to have your pets in your room, I always prefer that they sleep on their bed. If your pets are used to sleeping with you, I know it's hard to change this. Consider this a possible change since they are not the source of your insomnia but they may add to it when they move into your bed. On the other side, I also know pets can be comforting.

Read the labels of your personal care products, laundry, and dish detergent, and cleaning products; EWG Skin Deep has reviewed over ninety thousand products, so EWG is a good resource to check if the products you use are free of chemicals or not and what to choose in the future (Environmental Working Group 2023a).

EWG gives you access to the National Tap Water Database. You can use your zip code to check what chemicals are in the tap water in your area. Companies such as Doctors Data do water analysis if you want more detailed information. Use the guide from the EWG website to decide on a water filter that works for you.

If your car is newer or still smells like a new car when you enter, always air it out when you get in, especially when it's hot, and use a small USB air purifier in your vehicle while in your car.

Eat organic foods whenever possible, especially animal products, and check out the EWG "dirty dozen" and "clean fifteen" for fruits and vegetables, which is updated each year.

Reduce or altogether avoid fish that is high in mercury, such as tuna and swordfish since larger fish tend to accumulate more heavy metals, and shellfish. Stick to eating fish that are smaller, such as sardines. When you buy food that is not organic, wash it with fruit and vegetable wash to diminish some of the pesticides you ingest.

Avoid using herbicides on your lawn or garden. Remember that living on a golf course or playing golf increases your exposure significantly.

Avoid heating your car in the garage if your garage is underneath your bedroom, or park your car outside. Gas chemicals can off-gas and reach your bedroom.

Hire an EMF consultant to check EMF levels in your house; this may be a significant issue for some individuals.

Work with a biological dentist to see whether you have amalgam fillings, a source of heavy metals exposure, and/or cavitations from root canals. Cavitations are not the same as cavities. They are lesions within the jawbone due to blood flow blockage.

Clean up your environment at work as much as possible with the steps above, wherever applicable.

What do I do next?

Kidney detox support

Drink appropriate amounts of clean water to keep your kidneys in the best shape. The kidneys use water to eliminate some of the water-soluble toxins. You may determine the approximate right amount of water, including herbal teas, by dividing your weight by half; the number in ounces is how much you should consume daily. For example, if you are 150 pounds, you should drink around seventy-five ounces of water daily.

I like to sip on my water throughout the day instead of chugging it so it gets used better instead of immediately being eliminated through my bladder. If you drink bottled water, be aware that plastics may be leaking into your water.

The kidneys are considered second to the liver for detoxification. Toxins are made water-soluble in the liver and then excreted through the kidneys. The kidneys can effectively extract toxins from the blood, but if they are sluggish, toxic levels can accumulate in the kidneys, which will cause more damage to these organs.

Cadmium is a metal that affects the kidneys the most, with an extremely long half-life of ten years, so this is a critical metal to address to optimize kidney function. Other toxins that are excreted through the kidneys are mercury, lead, pesticides, herbicides, non-stick coatings, and fire retardants found in mattresses (Pizzorno 2015, 8-13).

A healthy diet with plenty of vegetables, especially beets, dandelion greens, parsley, celery, and asparagus, can support kidney health. Temporarily reduce animal protein, except fish, intake during this detox period. Eat fruits such as grapes, blueberries, and cranberries that support kidney detoxification. A supportive herbal combination to support your kidney function may include hydrangea, cranberry, alfalfa, rhodiola, and parsley.

Sweating to encourage detox

Sweating is another wonderful avenue for the water-soluble toxins to be eliminated (Sears, Kerr and Bray 2012, 1-10). Sweating can be done in an infrared sauna or through exercise, such as hot yoga. Strenuous exercise can also cause sweating but remember that if you are not sleeping well and already have imbalanced cortisol levels, strenuous exercise may not be the best strategy for recovery, at least to begin with.

Mild to moderate exercise will help with the detox process. It will create movement in your body and encourage lymph drainage to process unwanted toxins. Exercise also supports the kidneys' natural detox function. A study showed that women who exercised reduced kidney stones and improved bone strength (New York Daily News 2013).

Bowel movement regulation for detox

Ensure you have one to three bowel movements per day. Toxins get reabsorbed when bowel movement frequency slows down. Bowel movement may be slow for many reasons, such as inadequate water intake, stress, not enough exercise, too much dairy consumption, food sensitivities, travel, not listening to your body's urges and waiting to use the bathroom, insufficient fiber in your diet, imbalanced gut flora, low thyroid, IBS, and more severe issues such as colon cancer. Bowel movement is crucial because heavy metals such as mercury, lead, and cadmium are processed through the bile and eliminated in the stool.

Here are some things to consider about your bowel movement and how to ensure healthy elimination. Ensure you have enough fiber in your diet to encourage regular bowel movements. I recommend thirty to thirty-five grams. The American Heart Association recommends twenty-five to thirty grams while most Americans consume less than fifteen grams (McManus 2019). Fiber content can be increased by ensuring the most significant part of your plate is vegetables. Other fiber sources are fruits, eaten with the skin on, beans, nuts, and seeds including flaxseeds and chia seeds.

Many people are deficient in magnesium and can benefit from supplementing with it to promote healthy bowel movement. Magnesium citrate is the most laxative along with ozonated magnesium, which acts mainly on improving gut motility. Fiber supplementation, such as psyllium husk, can also be taken to improve bowel movement and healthy bacteria in your gut. Avoid Metamucil, a psyllium fiber supplement, because it has food coloring, which can affect some people negatively.

Lymphatic system support for detox

Your lymphatic system carries immune cells and helps flush out toxins. While the lymphatic system is directly connected to the cardiovascular system, it doesn't have an organ like the heart to keep the fluids going.

Gravity stimulates lymph; hello, inversions, head stands, and arm stands. Only do them if you can safely do so. The lymph is also stimulated by muscle contraction, so movement is gold. Dry brushing can also increase lymph movement; use a dry brush and lightly use brushing strokes toward your heart. For even better results, use it before going in the sauna. Alternating cold and hot water showers can encourage lymph movement.

Lymph drainage therapy is a form of massage that is highly effective in increasing lymph movement.

You may have heard of the *glymphatic system*—the lymphatic system of the brain and spinal cord, which clears out byproducts and toxins. This lymphatic movement happens most effectively if we sleep enough and support the other main detox pathways.

In addition, deep breathing helps encourage lymph movement throughout the body, including the glymphatic system.

Liver detox and support

The liver, with its three phases of detoxification, is the most important organ when it comes to processing toxins and preparing them for elimination. The bile from the gallbladder also plays a role in the detox process. One of the best ways to support the liver is by simply eating healthier and decreasing exposure to toxins.

Herbs such as milk thistle, dandelion, and turmeric heal the liver; these are often combined with bitters, which help bile production, liver function, and bowel movement motility.

Bitter tinctures typically include herbs such as gentian, dandelion, burdock, and orange peel. The use of bitters or herbals that help stimulate the liver and gallbladder, and hence the elimination of toxins, are typically followed by a binder. Quicksilver Scientific has a product called Push and Catch that supports these processes.

Glutathione is naturally produced in the liver. It is a wonderful antioxidant and helps detox. N-acetyl cysteine is a precursor of glutathione and can be helpful as well.

The liver loves cruciferous vegetables such as broccoli, broccoli sprouts, brussels sprouts, cauliflower, cabbage, arugula, bok choy, and collard greens. Chicken or beef liver can also support your liver function. You can cook a wonderful chicken liver pate, which seems tastier than beef for some people, with onion, ghee or butter, fresh thyme, and salt and pepper; blend it and serve it on a rice cracker or gluten-free bread. Or have as-is.

If you don't have a gallbladder, taking TUDCA (Tauroursodeoxycholic acid), a bile acid derivative is helpful to aid digestion.

The use of binders to support detox

Binders such as activated charcoal can trap toxins and move them along in the bowel movement to be eliminated effectively. They are commonly used along with liver detoxification protocols.

Fulvic acid, which comes from humic acid found in dirt,

is a binder that can be used to remove metals and other toxins from your body.

Zeolite is another binder commonly used along with silica.

Most of the binders can also bind onto healthy nutrients, which is why understanding how to use them is crucial. Binders should always be ingested away from food or other supplements on an empty stomach.

Apple pectin is a natural binder that does not attach to healthy nutrients in your body. Note that different binders work for various toxins, so appropriate help is needed to identify which toxins are high in your body, via testing, and which binders are recommended. Consult with a practitioner before adding this supplement regimen.

Eating to detox

Eating mindfully to encourage healthy elimination and optimizing the various organs that we've talked about so far is the gentlest and best way to support metabolic detoxification.

Start with the standard elimination diet to eliminate gluten-containing foods, dairy, eggs, corn, soy, alcohol, sugar, and caffeine for two months. This diet is usually done for one month, but when detox is the purpose, I choose a longer-term approach such as two months, to give the body a real break from possible stressors.

Focus on a daily diet that includes high amounts of vegetables and fruits:

- Two cups of green leafy vegetables
- Two cups of diversely colored non-starchy vegetables
- Two cups of fruit

These fresh fruits and vegetables will give you ample nutrients in their whole form to provide you with all you need to detox.

Colorful fruits and vegetables provide wonderful phytonutrients that are highly anti-oxidative and anti-inflammatory—basically, eat the rainbow every day.

Starchy vegetables can also be used to help detox. They are lovely because they offer quick energy; however, they are best eaten in a complete meal (or snack) that includes protein and fat for stable blood sugar.

If the increased amount of vegetables causes loose stools or you have trouble digesting them, choose to cook most or all of them lightly. I see this as the better choice anyway, as many of us have what we in Chinese medicine call "diminished digestive fire," where we have a hard time breaking down food that has not been at least lightly cooked.

We need good quality protein to detox, so use small amounts of beans that have been soaked or sprouted for one serving per day, grass-fed beef, organic chicken, and fish such as salmon, sardines, or mackerel.

Collagen powders from grass-fed beef or fish sources can provide the protein macronutrient for a breakfast smoothie, soup, or snack.

Use seeds and nuts that have been soaked. Check online for proper soaking times. Use healthy fats such as coconut products, olive oil, avocado oil and fresh avocado, and flaxseed oil.

Grains are kept low in this diet; some acceptable ones would be quinoa (a seed), buckwheat, rice, and millet.

Dandelion root tea is one of my favorite drinks, which resembles the coffee taste, to help detox. You can use spices and condiments freely, and they are highly encouraged. Turmeric, rosemary, ginger, and pepper are some of my favorites.

Refer to the GI chapter for the reintroduction of foods after two months of this diet and work with a practitioner to get the best results.

Detoxing safely

People can easily get more ill when trying to detox by themselves, which is why I always recommend that you do it with the help of a professional. Optimizing your water intake, improving your diet for a better bowel movement, and eating a cleaner diet are likely steps that can be done on your own.

Step-by-step action items

- As you read this chapter, take note of areas where you can reduce exposure to toxins at home, in your car, and at work.
- Replace items whenever possible.
- Invest in an air purifier.
- Support your kidneys, lymphatic system, and liver detox process.
- Work with your diet to help your body detox.
- Work with a practitioner to get additional support through testing and treatment.

CHAPTER TWELVE

CHRONIC INFECTIONS AND BIOTOXINS

The aim of this chapter

- Understand what may be at the root of chronic complex insomnia.
- Understand how chronic infections and biotoxin toxicity are affecting your health.
- Get an overview of EBV (Epstein-Barr virus), Lyme disease, mold toxicity, mast cell activation, and more.
- Receive step-by-step guidance on what to do next with these complex issues.

The world of chronic infections is a complicated one. My patients come in because they can't sleep. They are telling themselves that if they could just sleep, all would be well.

Unfortunately, the effects of these rather complex syndromes are varied, and sleeping well is just one part of the healing process.

Along with chronic infections, we will discuss biotoxin toxicity, particularly mold. The symptoms are multi-system, just like with the toxic burden. People may experience fatigue, brain fog, insomnia, depression, anxiety, neurological symptoms, GI symptoms, muscle pain, and more.

For some people, this illness escalates to the point where it goes into CIRS—chronic inflammatory response syndrome. The body is basically under attack and has to respond accordingly—all in the name of survival.

Why chronic infections and biotoxins are factors in sleep issues

Chronic infections and biotoxin exposure can cause a heightened immune system response, which sets off cascades of inflammation. This cascade can result in two other possible health consequences: MCAS (mast cell activation syndrome) and/or MCS (multiple chemical sensitivity).

In general terms, MCAS tends to be triggered more specifically by foods we eat where MCS tends to be triggered by environmental toxins such as smells of perfumes, detergent, and so on.

The depleted and the overburdened types often struggle with the issues presented in this chapter. Typical therapies don't tend to work, or if they work, don't hold.

Some practitioners are not trained to understand the root cause of these issues. Since many systems are affected, such as the stress response, hormones, and gastrointestinal disorders, some practitioners will do as I have done: keep working on specific systems such as hormones, stress response, and the like, which of course, is only helpful to a degree for many people. We need to find the constant trigger (or triggers) to make real progress in our health.

There are many types of biotoxins, but as mentioned earlier, we will be talking about mold toxicity. When referring to chronic infections, the focus will be more specifically on EBV (Epstein-Barr virus), Lyme, co-infections, and parasites.

Most people are likely never to develop problems from toxins such as mold. However, some people have genetic variants in the human leukocyte antigen (HLA) gene complex and don't have a proper immune response to mold (Valtonen 2017).

Healthy inflammation leads to the activation of cytokines —small proteins that help guide the inflammatory process. They are like a healthy, contained fire. But when the inflammatory process overloads due to high toxicity and an inability to control the virus or toxin, it evolves into a scary, giant, biochemically uncontrolled fire. Sleeping, under those circumstances, is not ideal. The body is under a red alert.

For example, when you have a virus like influenza (the flu), your sleep is terrible at night, but thankfully you may be able to sleep during the day. Plus the illness is short-lived.

With biotoxins and chronic infections, people suffer for months and years; hence, the chronic nature of the sleep issues and why taking some melatonin and valerian, for example, rarely makes a dent. People take one, two, or even three sleep medications and many herbs or supplements in these situations. Yet, sleep is elusive.

Let's expose how this disease process affects the body, so we can understand how to approach healing this chronic type of insomnia.

Assessing for chronic infections and mold toxicity

Some of the most common infections that may cause chronic diseases are often called "silent" infections because they don't always have symptoms that point toward an obvious cause, infection, or diagnosis. Instead, people start feeling unwell, develop autoimmune disorders, or experience a wide range of symptoms that don't fit any particular disease profile.

These infections affect different systems in various ways. In time they will depress the immune system and create inflammation. The overburdened type often struggles with chronic infections, especially when feeling ill. The other insomnia types may also struggle with an infection or two from this list.

What also tends to happen with the following chronic infections is that people feel worse cyclically. They have periods when they tend to feel better, their sleep improves, and then they feel worse for no particular reason.

Note that insomnia can also be cyclical in menstruating women during the premenstrual phase, generally one week before your bleeding starts.

Although you may be familiar with some of these infections from prior chapters, here is an expanded list. Common chronic infections that people struggle with:

- Epstein-Barr Virus (EBV)
- Candida and other fungal overgrowth, such as mold
- Lyme disease and other spirochetes
- *Blastocystis hominis*, *Chilomastix mesnili*, and other parasites
- Overgrowth of commensal bacteria *Clostridioides*

- Overgrowth of *H. pylori*
- Cytomegalovirus (CMV)
- Bacteria associated with stealthy dental abscesses and infections, or cavitations

We will focus on the first four in more depth since there seems to be more of a common association with sleep issues in my clinical practice, though this does not mean that the other chronic infections could not be related or contributing to your insomnia. Some of these are covered in other chapters in this book; others you will have to explore with your health care professional.

Assessing for chronic infections and biotoxin toxicity requires the help of a medical professional. This chapter helps you identify if this is what may be happening in your body. Then, being more informed, you will likely find the right practitioner to understand your symptoms and do some testing.

Working with a knowledgeable practitioner is essential since the world of mold toxicity, EBV, and Lyme disease with its co-infections is not only a specialty but also one that is not fully understood and standardized in the medical community. It is an emerging and evolving field regarding diagnosis and treatments.

If you recognize yourself within this chapter, look for health practitioners who are literate in the world of issues related to mold, Lyme disease, EBV, etc.

Each case is different, but many patients require medications, herbs, and supplements to heal. So find a practitioner with prescribing authority or, if not, a practitioner who works closely with a prescribing doctor. For example, many naturopaths specialize in these illnesses and often work closely with medical doctors who can prescribe medications if needed.

Cell danger response

Before diving into more specifics, it is crucial to grasp a vital concept coined by Dr. Robert Naviaux: *cell danger response* (Naviaux 2014, 7-17). Once there is an attack or stressor, the powerhouses of our body, mitochondria, shift part of their function from producing energy to defense mode.

However, if the stressor is ongoing or the body has specific genetic weaknesses, it will get stuck in that stress mode.

There are three stages to this cell danger response. Each process is an opportunity to return to the healthy healing process, and restorative sleep is one factor that influences the ability to do so instead of being stuck in defense and inflammation mode.

This process of the cell danger response means the chronic disease can often develop due to the *reaction* to the initial injury rather than the injury itself. That is why the terrain is so important: How resilient are we under trauma, a stressor, or a toxin? Our resilience differs based on many factors—from our overall state of health, genetics, age, other chronic illness, and more. It can also depend on whether there is a repeat injury before the first one can heal.

What we notice with chronic disease is that it becomes a *system* disease instead of an isolated acute illness or disease that can focus more on one particular area or system of the body. That's why we have to work holistically and with an integrated approach when it comes to chronic disease.

One supplement, one herb, or one medication is rarely able to help your insomnia to heal fully. Chronic insomnia is a symptom of more significant issues, likely due to a system or multiple systems dysfunction.

Patients with chronic disease, and especially with disorders presented in this chapter, struggle with fatigue. Since my patients all suffer from insomnia, the general idea is that if I could sleep, I would feel so much better. In some people, restoring their sleep improves their energy during the day, either because sleep deprivation was the main reason for the fatigue and/or because restorative sleep improves other bodily functions.

However, I have worked with a subset of people in my practice whose sleep improves, yet they are still fatigued. Low energy is present because something else still affects energy production. In many cases, it is the need to address this mitochondrial function. There are other reasons for fatigue, such as hypothyroidism, sleep apnea, and more. However, mold toxicity and chronic infections are high on the list for my patients struggling with profound, relentless fatigue, especially when unresolved after sleeping better.

A straightforward example of the mitochondria shifting their focus toward defense is when we are exposed to a virus like influenza (the flu). The intense achiness and fatigue that comes with it can be seen as a protective mechanism to slow down. But this fatigue is also an effect of the mitochondria shifting focus toward defense rather than energy production.

In addition, the symptoms are not caused directly by the virus but rather from the body's reaction *to it*. The mobilization of immune markers leads to the symptoms we feel. Just as with chronic illnesses, the response to the trigger causes the cascade that leads to chronic disease, not the initial trauma. Of course, the inflammatory markers will also be ongoing if there are continuing triggers such as allergic food, mold exposure, or an active infection.

This cell danger response mechanism is why there are two critical steps in healing chronic disease:

- identifying and removing any perpetrators like chronic stress, poor diet, viruses, mold, etc.
- helping the body get out of the automatic stress response that it has been stuck on—sometimes for years.

Reactivated Epstein-Barr Virus (EBV)

EBV is a virus present in over 98 percent of the human population. EBV is the virus responsible for causing mononucleosis. It is also called the "kissing disease," as it can be easily transmitted through saliva. Some people can be sick for a few weeks; in rare cases, it can take up to six months to recover.

After the recovery, the virus lies dormant in the body and can be reactivated when the immune system is weakened. The longer the recovery from the mononucleosis, the more likely the virus may get reactivated later. This long recovery period shows the immune system having difficulty with the initial infection, which may imply a more challenging time keeping it in control later throughout life.

The main symptom of chronic EBV infection is fatigue. It may also show up with chronic sore throat, swollen glands, anxiety, or a chronically slightly elevated fever. Reactivated EBV can often be seen in people who also have Lyme disease. EBV may be connected to the development of certain autoimmune disorders (National Institutes of Health 2018).

The reactivated EBV is essential when it comes to sleep because it tends to affect the body over time in various ways. It can affect the function of neurotransmitters, the sympathetic nervous system, and it can negatively impact cortisol levels. It increases inflammatory markers affecting the body overall, which causes an activated stress response and insomnia. It may also affect your sleep by altering gut function, which can keep you up because it causes your body temperature to be slightly elevated.

Unfortunately, some of my patients who struggle with chronic, intractable insomnia are sometimes diagnosed with various issues in addition to EBV, such as mold toxicity and Lyme. It is scary to hear this, but it is reassuring when we understand the basic principles: We don't treat the disease but ultimately the immune system.

The standard markers used in the medical community are EBV-VCA IgG, EBV-VCA IgM, and EBV nuclear antigen antibodies (ENBA). A fourth marker is often missed and only tested when throat cancer is suspected. Early Antigen Antibodies IgG is typically high in new infections, but for some people is reactivated later. This marker tells us that the virus is actively replicating; therefore, it is essential to test when checking for EBV infection and possible reactivation.

Use laboratories that give you the results in numbers instead of "negative" or "positive" results. The exact numbers for each marker are helpful in understanding the clinical picture for a knowledgeable practitioner who is keeping a healing systems approach in mind.

Mold toxicity

Mold exposure and toxicity are a lot more common than we think. If you have the genetic variant that makes you less able to clear this toxicity, you are unfortunately more likely to get sick. Some people are aware of being exposed to a moldy environment. But many others are completely unaware of it. It may be hiding in a wall, swamp cooler, or a closet. It might not be visible to the naked eye, and we might not even be able to smell it, or if we do, we become used to it and cannot identify it as a musty or moldy smell.

People have two types of reactions to mold:

- Some people have an allergic reaction, an IgE reaction of the immune system that usually leads to asthma and allergies as the main symptoms.
- The second possible reaction is mold sensitivity, which is less understood by the medical community but is nonetheless the cause of health struggles for many people. In this case, the body cannot eliminate the mold toxins properly, and the mold colonizes in places such as the sinuses, lungs, or the GI system.

Here are some things to look for from observing your environment or the symptoms you are experiencing if you suspect mold toxicity:

- You notice apparent mold growth in spaces you live in, work in, or visit.
- You live or work in a place that has been flooded for more than twelve hours.
- You have been or are exposed to a place that has a "musty" smell.
- You have been exposed to mold and have felt unwell since.
- You notice you are gradually sensitive to more foods, despite a good diet.
- You are more susceptible to your environment, smells, etc.

- You do not respond well or at all to medications for your symptoms.
- You have been to numerous doctors, and the treatments make little difference.

Three particular symptoms that Dr. Neil Nathan talks about in his book *Toxic: Heal Your Body from Mold Toxicity, Lyme Disease, Multiple Chemical Sensitivities, and Chronic Environmental Illness* should have you immediately explore the possibility of mold-related illness are:

1. electric shock sensations
2. ice-pick like pains
3. vibrating or pulsating sensations up and down the spine (Nathan 2018, 40)

You may experience (especially initially) a runny nose, sneezing, asthma, cough, bloating, abdominal pain, loose stools, or diarrhea. These symptoms will persist, or with some people, they morph into chronic sinus issues, brain fog, memory issues, fatigue, insomnia, anxiety, neurological symptoms, headaches, joint pain, urination problems, or eye problems and sensitivities.

Once you assess that mold colonization may be the root of why you are unwell, it is time to take the next step. The assessment usually requires a combination of approaches.

First, check your suspected environment for mold through an ERMI test. You can order this test online and have it shipped to your house. You collect a sample, mail it back to the lab, and get results within a week. You will need separate kits for your home, office, or other environments. Nearly all mold toxicity comes from indoors; outdoor molds usually don't trigger an illness, but once ill, they could be a source of aggravation.

Do a visual contrast sensitivity test (VCS). This is an affordable test for optic nerve inflammation that can be done online. A failed test may be associated with a high indication of a biotoxin, not precisely mold, but still helpful. Note that this is not a diagnostic test but another one that may help with the bigger clinical picture. The failed VCS test, in combination with a positive mold questionnaire, can show a high likelihood of mold toxicity, according to Dr. Ritchie Shoemaker, an expert in this field (Surviving Mold, n.d.).

NeuroQuant is a type of MRI that shows changes in the brain due to biotoxins, such as mold.

A series of blood tests can show chronic inflammation, such as MSH, ADH/osmolality, ACTH/cortisol, MMP-9, and C4a.

Genetic testing for *HLA-DRB1, 3, 4, and 5* can show if you are among the individuals who have more trouble detoxing mold than the rest of the population.

A urine mycotoxin test is often useful; however, some people can be in a highly toxic state with the body unable to excrete toxins since excreting would make the toxins more available in the circulation and aggravate the illness, and the urine markers would show negative. That is when working with a practitioner and looking at the bigger picture will help you identify if mold is part of what is making you ill.

Another test to identify whether mold is making you sick is a blood test that assesses whether there is an immune reaction to certain molds. One of the companies providing such tests is Cyrex Laboratory, specifically Array 12.

MARCoNS

Patients with mold exposure and a weakened immune system may have bacterial colonization in the sinus called MARCoNS (Multiple Antibiotic Resistant Coagulase Negative Staphylococci).

This colonization produces its toxin, called *exotoxin A*, which further weakens the immune system. So treating this infection is crucial in the treatment of mold toxicity.

Testing for this nasal bacterial and fungal infection is done by a nasal swab, and the treatment is specific nasal sprays and/or antibiotics.

Lyme disease and co-infections

The first time I read about how the infection from a tick gets transmitted, I was fascinated. When a tick bites you, it draws a bit of your blood into its stomach, takes twelve to twenty-four hours to mix it up with its own "juices," and then injects this toxic mixture into your body. This mixture may include a rather complex cocktail: the bacteria *Borrelia,* which causes Lyme disease, the bacteria *Bartonella*, which is commonly found in people who also have mold toxicity, the parasite *Babesia*, and the microbes *Ehrlichia*, *Anaplasma*, and *Rickettsia*. Unfortunately, these organisms can all live within the same tick. Hence a person can be infected with more than one at a time.

How do we identify whether we have been infected with Lyme disease and its co-infections? Here is what to look for. If a tick bite is followed by headaches, fatigue, and a skin rash called *erythema*, seek help from your doctor.

The main symptoms that come from Lyme disease are neurological and joint/muscle related: muscle and joint pain, fatigue, poor sleep, mental fogginess and decreased ability to concentrate, and nerve pain.

Some of the main symptoms that come from a *Bartonella* infection are intense anxiety and panic attacks, insomnia, a sensation of vibration in the body—note that this feeling is most common with feeling wired in the evening due to high cortisol, often found outside of this infection—GI symptoms, joint pain, pelvic pain, and neurological symptoms.

The third main co-infection is the parasite *Babesia;* some of the symptoms that can show up are night sweats, "air hunger," feeling like you can't take a deep breath despite standard oxygen saturation numbers, and a hard time focusing on tasks and performing them.

Lyme disease and its co-infections can lie dormant for months or years without obvious symptoms. Likely when the immune system is weakened by something else—such as chronic stress, mold exposure, perimenopause, or a car accident—Lyme disease becomes symptomatic.

Identifying if Lyme disease is the culprit is more complex than we would like it to be. Here are some things to consider:

- The standard test to check for Lyme disease is the Western blot blood test; however, this test yields a high rate of false negatives so consider finding practitioners who use specialty labs such as IGeneX.
- The VCS test in the mold section can indicate possible Lyme disease and co-infections. The questionnaire with the test asks questions related to mold and tick-borne diseases.

- The NeuroQuant scan can also detect changes in the brain due to Lyme and co-infection toxicity.
- Finally, the Horowitz Lyme-MSIDS Questionnaire is also used to pinpoint many Lyme disease-related symptoms.

CIRS—chronic inflammatory response syndrome

The more significant concern with biotoxin toxicity and its effects on the body is that these symptoms can further develop into CIRS—chronic inflammatory response syndrome. In CIRS, the immune system is like a raging fire, as explained earlier in this chapter. It's out of control because it cannot remove the toxicity that started the process. For example, mold accumulates in the body because no antibodies to these biotoxins are produced in genetically susceptible people. See the online genetics chapter.

Here are a few things to consider as causes of CIRS. It may be due to exposure to water-damaged buildings and the consequences of inhaling mold spores and subsequent colonization and other biotoxins exposure. Tick or spider bites, which you may or may not have been aware of, may lead to the transmission of *Borrelia*, *Bartonella*, *Babesia*, etc., and can cause CIRS.

If you have gotten sick from eating fish, the fish could have been contaminated with dinoflagellate algae, some of which produce Ciguatera toxin, which has been associated with CIRS. Water contamination exposure to toxins in areas of fish kills, such as *Pfiesteria* and *Cyanobacteria* is also another possible cause.

In healthy individuals who don't have a genetic susceptibility, exposure to these will likely lead to the body recognizing these biotoxins, binding them, and excreting them out through the stool. In the susceptible individual, these biotoxins go from cell to cell, creating damage that triggers a whole host of immune responses.

The immune response becomes chronic, and the inflammation response accelerates. Multiple systems are affected, and the person suffers from many complaints, with most remedies unable to offer relief since the root problem is not solved.

People with CIRS are frequently diagnosed with some of the following diseases: chronic fatigue syndrome, fibromyalgia, IBS, PTSD, ADD, ADHD, allergies, anxiety, depression, and insomnia. The symptoms that tend to come with this syndrome are varied and complex. Hence it is somewhat confusing and hard to pinpoint where the root problem is.

Mast cell activation syndrome (MCAS) & multiple chemical sensitivity (MCS)

In simple terms, most MCAS is triggered by what you eat and drink, and MCS is started by what you smell.

Most patients who have biotoxin toxicity and develop MCAS likely also have insomnia. This is because the mast cells are the connection between the immune system and the nervous system. Frequently the person who struggles with so many symptoms is referred to a psychiatrist. All of these symptoms, it is thought, must be psychosomatic! Patients are often incredibly frustrated, understandably.

Mast cells are part of the immune system, though not as well-known as white blood cells. Their job is to deal with toxins and infectious agents; therefore, the highest numbers are found in tissues close to the outside world—sinuses, throat, gastrointestinal tract, skin, respiratory tract, and genito-urinary tract. They are filled with *granules* with potential energy that stimulates histamine, serotonin, and tryptase production.

When overstimulated by toxicity, mast cells start overreacting to foods, drinks, scents, chemicals, etc. In extreme situations, someone could react strongly to a glass of water.

When activated, a lot more histamines are released in the body. High histamine or histamine intolerance causes insomnia because histamine acts as an excitatory neurotransmitter, which is why Benadryl can help people sleep because of its antihistamine function.

A different scenario that can surface is becoming very sensitive to chemicals and triggering what we call MCS. MCS may feel similar to MCAS; however, MCS tends to be triggered by what we inhale rather than eat. According to Dr. Neil Nathan, it is rare for an individual to have MCS and not have mold toxicity.

Typical MCS symptoms tend to worsen after exposure and persist for hours or days. The person may experience headaches, mental exhaustion, neurological disorders, such as tics and tremors, and dizziness. The most common symptom associated with MCS is anxiety.

It is hard to be anywhere except the patient's residence since everything may feel like a trigger. The nervous system is alert and reacts strongly to even the faintest exposure. These patients tend to be highly sensitive to any EMF exposure. They tend to respond strongly to therapies, supplements, or medications; they feel very "sensitive" to anything they take.

Parasites and sleep

Parasites are organisms that feed on other organisms to survive and thrive. Parasites can be passed through food or water, especially in underdeveloped countries, contaminated vegetables or fruit, or undercooked fish or meat. They can also be found in creeks, ponds, and lakes.

Some of the symptoms you may experience if you have parasites are: grinding your teeth while you sleep, trouble falling asleep or staying asleep, sleep talking, gastrointestinal symptoms that are unexplained, such as IBS symptoms, skin problems, achy joints, never felt well since you had food poisoning, and iron-deficiency anemia.

The parasite will activate the immune system and may raise cortisol levels. In addition, parasites can produce ammonia, which may affect glutamate and GABA levels and therefore sleep.

Blastocystis hominis is seen in some studies concerning sleep disorders and is also present with autoimmune disorders; it is a contributor in other diseases such as chronic urticaria, itching, and GERD (Wedi 2009, 10; El-Zawawy and Farag 2020).

Some parasites cause insomnia because of the itching and irritation at night; some examples are *Cyclospora cayetanensis, Dientamoeba fragilis*, and *Trichuris. Ancylostoma duodenale* is associated with sleep issues (Babatunde et al. 2013, 2613-2317; Vezir 2019 927-932).

Stool tests can identify parasites, but some tests have limited capabilities or low sensitivity to parasites.

However, a comprehensive stool test is an excellent place to start. Some companies, such as Doctor's Data, do a three-day stool sample, which has a higher probability of identifying a parasite in the stool. PCR testing (such as GI Map) looks for a number of specific parasites in the stool. Other companies offer comprehensive stool tests such as Genova Diagnostics Laboratory and Vibrant Wellness.

Healing your chronic infections and mold toxicity to heal your sleep

I have worked with patients who have mold toxicity, Lyme disease and co-infections, and reactivated EBV—all of this leading to CIRS. To top things off, some develop MCAS, which makes intake of food complicated as they have no idea what they are reacting to.

Then they can't even go out in the world, as they may sense a perfume smell and get a migraine. In this case, the entire being is in a state of fight or flight, with an incredibly high sensitivity to almost everything.

This all happens in the name of a protective mechanism in the body. The body says, we are so over the edge, we cannot afford any more attackers, or all will be lost. So we will react to everything—almost all foods, all smells, any stimulants. The resilience is not there anymore.

Your entire being feels like a severely abused child; we have to take it easy, be gentle, build trust, go slow, and not stop when there are setbacks. Just be there and just learn from them. And keep going. Because we are capable of incredible healing.

Prepare the foundation for healing

As much as you want to get going to get rid of the mold or kill the EBV or Lyme infection, your body may not have the resources or be ready for that. Your body is likely stuck in defense mode, and every aspect of your immune system focuses on that defense.

Strengthening the body with nourishing nutrition and calming the nervous system is crucial. Working on supporting your depleted and tired immune system is also impactful. All this can happen before using antiviral or antibiotic herbs and drugs, binders for mycotoxins, or antifungals. These agents can be potent and sometimes "kill" more than we would like them to, making us feel even sicker.

Improving your diet to get stronger

You may already be eating healthy; you may suffer from food sensitivities, and working on your diet may seem complicated. Because of your ongoing health issues and insomnia, your cortisol levels are likely imbalanced throughout the day and night.

Here are some simple steps to get you going to get stronger:

- If you've never done the elimination diet that I have recommended throughout the book to support gut health, consider doing so now. Eliminate some or all foods for four weeks: gluten, eggs, dairy, corn, soy, alcohol, and sugar. Sugar, which can come from too many carbs, sweets, or alcohol, can numb the immune system. Sugar puts the immune cells in a temporary coma for about five hours (Sanchez et al. 1973, 1180-1184).

- Eat two cups of green leafy vegetables per day. Don't cheat. Push those leaves so it's a full cup. Add in two cups of colorful veggies, and two cups of fruit. As you get better and better at this, you may add another cup of colorful veggies and green leafy vegetables. The more fresh vegetables and fruits you eat along with healthy protein and fat, the more you get essential nutrients for healing. Soups and smoothies may be a simpler way to incorporate this increased vegetable intake.
- Eat three times daily; do your best to make them all complete meals with all macronutrients—carbs, protein, and fat.
- Use the adrenal diet. Eat within one hour of waking and get steady nutrition throughout the day.

Supplementing the core nutrients

You are building on a healthier diet, so nourishing supplements is the next step:

- Vitamin D is crucial for immune response; always test before supplementing with a blood test. People's needs vary widely depending on altitude, sun exposure, sunscreen use, and genetics. Optimal levels are sixty to eighty ng/ml. The active form of vitamin D is D3.
- Omega-3 support through fish oil, such as liver cod oil, will provide a highly absorbable amount of vitamins A and D and can drastically reduce inflammation. Work with your practitioner on the EPA/DHA ratio based on your needs.
- Take Vitamin C in the liposomal form to support the immune system and because it stimulates bile production,

which can help eliminate mold; a standard dose is five hundred milligrams, twice daily.

- Supplement with probiotics and prebiotic powder to support gut function to improve the immune system.
- The secretory IgA, the gut immune system, is often significantly depleted, so taking bovine-based immunoglobulins can support the immune system.
- Magnesium is a cofactor needed for many different functions in the body. It is a support for anxiety, stress, and insomnia relief. Some of the best forms of magnesium are magnesium threonate, since it passes the blood-brain barrier, and magnesium glycinate, which will systemically affect the whole body.
- Curcumin is a potent anti-inflammatory and the active and principal ingredient in turmeric, so taking curcumin is more powerful than just taking turmeric.
- For HPA axis support, refer to the stress response chapter.

EBV healing

In addition to all the steps presented above, some herbs and supplements have antiviral properties. Remember that healing EBV takes time. While it's helpful to use antiviral agents, it is equally important to lower stress and increase your immune system's ability to keep this virus in check. Remember that the virus never goes away; it just stays dormant and no longer actively replicates.

Some valuable supplements and herbs to support the healing process include L-lysine, monolaurin, Chinese skullcap, frankincense, and reishi mushrooms.

One of the books that dive deep into this virus is by the Doctor of Clinical Nutrition Dr. Kasia Kines, *The Epstein-Barr Virus Solution*. This extensive book has everything you must know to heal from this complex virus reactivation.

Mold toxicity healing

One of the most essential steps to heal mold toxicity is ensuring you are no longer exposed. If you have been exposed to mold in your home, you must remediate it. Some people need to move out of their homes.

Mold is a fungus, so it is helpful to eat an antifungal diet. Funguses feed on sugar. Remember, *Candida* overgrowth is fungal overgrowth. Many of my patients have elevated mycotoxins along with *Candida* overgrowth.

Test with organic acid and mycotoxin tests, work with a practitioner, and retest in three to six months.

Focus on a whole foods diet and minimize refined sugars, such as described above; do not avoid carbs and sugar altogether because the brain needs constant and quick energy to sleep well.

Avoid mold- and yeast-containing foods, such as cheese, alcohol, condiments, fungi, cured and smoked meats, dried fruits, and coffee. Look for mold-free coffee once you sleep better.

Invest in an air purifier; some brands claim that they can clear the room of mold spores. An air purifier is essential since even small amounts can make you sick until you detox. Also, even after remediation or if you've moved, mold can persist in small quantities, either because you are still in the remediated environment or because you may have brought some items contaminated with mold.

Use supplements such as glutathione, milk thistle, and NAC (N-Acetyl-Cysteine) to support the liver detox. To further enhance detox, use infrared saunas and dry brushing a minimum of two times per week until testing shows mold clearance.

Use antifungal supplements, herbs, or medication if needed. Use binders to help eliminate mycotoxins. Some binders are universal while others may be more specific, depending on the type of mold you are attempting to detox.

Cholestyramine is a medication that can be used as a binder for relatively short periods and is effective but can have moderately severe side effects for some people. Another one to consider with your doctor is Welchol.

And very importantly, ensure healthy, daily bowel movements.

Lyme disease and co-infection healing

Enter the wild world of healing Lyme disease and its co-infections. Yet again, I hope you are working with a practitioner on this one. The books *Healing Lyme* and *Healing Lyme Disease Co-infections* by Stephen Harrod Buhner are rich sources on the disease process and healing protocols that can be done (Buhner 2013; Buhner 2015).

In general, we aim to use an anti-inflammatory diet that supports the immune system, take antimicrobial herbs and pharmaceuticals whenever appropriate, and work on gut healing since these infections often affect the gut health. Always check for other possible issues, such as mold exposure, which I have seen go hand-in-hand with Lyme.

CIRS healing

The body's out-of-control inflammation, either due to mold or Lyme disease, causes many health problems for some people. This level of imbalance is where insomnia is genuinely a problem.

Find the root cause of why the inflammatory response got triggered—e.g., Lyme disease—and work on healing it to address CIRS.

Mast cell activation syndrome & multiple chemical sensitivity healing

As the mast cells are activated, histamines also get activated. A high histamine response is particularly troublesome if you have variants in the histamine genes, as presented in the online genetics chapter.

A low histamine diet can help move along the healing process along with supplements and herbs such as quercetin, watercress, chamomile, nettle tea or tincture, and curcumin.

If you suffer from MCS, address the exposures and work on the healing process step by step.

Parasite healing

Parasites can be directly correlated to nighttime awakenings. Each treatment may vary based on the particular parasite.

Blastocystis hominis can be addressed with the probiotic yeast *Saccharomyces boulardii;* one of the medications used for the short term to eradicate it is Alinia. This parasite is often not treated if the patient is not experiencing diarrhea; however, high growth is inflammatory and has been associated with autoimmune disorders (El-Zawawy and Farag 2020).

Other parasite treatments are done in two rounds of fourteen days with herbs such as walnut hull tincture, berberine, barberry, holy basil, and clove bud.

Bringing comfort

If you find yourself in this chapter, your health issues may be very stressful for you because of your symptoms or a previous diagnosis. Not sleeping, for any reason, is stressful. Not sleeping and suffering from mold toxicity or chronic infection is even worse.

The GI system is often affected. Remember that 70 percent of the immune system is located in the gut. Hormones often shift and change because of the stress response in the body. Stress is one of the leading known reasons for EBV reactivation.

How can we bring some comfort and set a baseline to lower the stress or at least manage the stress—real and perceived?

The sleep foundations chapter contains several ideas on implementing some routines and what could help your nervous system to calm down. When setting yourself up for months, if not longer, to truly heal, it helps to get clear on the light at the end of the tunnel and never lose sight of that goal. Otherwise, you will have a much harder time getting there.

Here is what I think about it. First, see if you can find a place in your mind, even if it's a tiny place, where you know, deep down, that healing is possible. I know it's hard, and you may have been at this for a while, but think about it this way: Who do you think you are that you cannot heal? It's a different way of looking at it, but again, why do you think you are no more or less "special" than the many people who do heal? Find something within your mind that portrays healing as possible; it may be an experience when something unexpected happened, faith in a higher power, or simply the deep desire to heal because you want to be healthy to be present for a loved one.

Next, what one thing can you do consistently in the morning and at night, no matter what, no matter how, that interrupts the stress response, reminds you of your breath, and helps you feel better? If not every day, five days a week.

- You could always take time for breakfast, and one minute before it, you close your eyes and breathe.
- You could take a hot shower every night, brush your teeth, sit in a chair with your eyes closed, and meditate or pray for ten minutes.
- Find that anchor in the morning and night, no matter the ups and downs. Stick with it. Refer to sleep foundations for many more ideas.

Who are your helpers? Because let's admit it: We need help, regardless of which insomniac type we are or which healing chapter we find ourselves in. But if this is more so your chapter, you need to find your helpers. Reliable helpers can be a combination of loved ones, a pet, a therapist, a yoga instructor, health coaches, and medical providers who will guide you through this process and see it through, even when it's hard.

Step-by-step action items

- Find a practitioner to help you identify the infection and/or biotoxin and support you through the healing stages.
- Address nutritional insufficiencies and work with lifestyle changes.
- Calm the sympathetic nervous system and activate the parasympathetic nervous system so you can start sleeping again by addressing the root issues and revisiting the stress response chapter.
- Encourage a healthy immune system response.
- Treat the infection or toxicity directly.

PART IV

SLEEP FOUNDATIONS

Part IV focuses on sleep foundations, which includes sleep hygiene, but it goes beyond into concepts I have found valuable in my clinical practice.

CHAPTER THIRTEEN

PREPARING FOR SLEEP

Clock or No Clock?

Before going into the sleep hygiene world, I want to discuss the alarm clock dilemma. A few points are crucial to facilitate the healing of insomnia.

Should we use an alarm clock? The short answer is yes. But the longer answer is more complicated. I like using an alarm clock in the morning as a backup. One of the stories I hear repeatedly is, "I don't need an alarm clock; I wake up by myself anyways. It would be a miracle if I didn't!"

I like using an alarm clock as a safety net. Since an alarm clock is set for the time you need to wake up, you have no need to glance at it in the middle of the night.

Avoiding clock-watching is key to the healing process. If you are awake for more than thirty minutes and want to know what time it is, that is fine. But barely waking up and checking the time within seconds or minutes is a recipe for worsening your sleep. Most of us have a sense of what time it is anyway. It typically feels very different if it's 2 a.m. instead of 5:30 a.m.

The moment we look at the clock, we start building a story. *Oh, it's 1:30 a.m., and I've only slept about three hours. If I don't fall asleep for another two hours, I probably won't be able to go back to sleep. I wonder what time it is now. It's 2:15; I still have plenty of time, maybe.* Sometime later, at 3 a.m., we are in a full-blown panic. *Tonight may be like one of those nights when I never go back to sleep.* And so it goes.

I am not saying the root of your insomnia is due to clock-watching, but checking the time may contribute to an exacerbation of your anxiety. If it's the middle of the night, it's not morning yet, so it doesn't matter what time it is. One of the few times when it does matter is if you are taking medication and need to count the number of hours left for next-day safety, but that is about it.

A clock you can immediately glance at fairly quickly must be moved or covered. I also recommend avoiding any radio-type alarm clock next to your bed since it's plugged in and likely emitting higher electrical fields than the earth's natural field. You may use your cell phone on airplane mode and not charging next to your bed or, even better, a battery-operated alarm clock that you have to touch for it to light up and show the time.

Most people who have their routine down tend to wake up at the same time. I still like the alarm clock idea, to let go completely and allow the mind to be as relaxed as possible, knowing it doesn't need to keep track of anything. I have found some patients sleeping deeper in the morning because of this. They realized that having no alarm clock set, they were vigilant about their morning.

The hour before sleep

The hour before sleep might be one of the most essential parts of this chapter.

Start by deciding on an ideal bedtime for you. It must be consistent, though it can vary slightly. I will explain why later in this chapter. To decide when to go to bed, you first determine your ideal wake-up time. Let's say it's 6 a.m. You count back either seven and a half or nine hours. If seven and a half hours sound good, bedtime will be 10:30 p.m.

If you have kids, your kids will change your plans some nights, and I understand that. But go with whatever would work in an ideal situation. Note that 10 p.m. to 2 a.m. is generally the more restorative sleep. This better sleep timeframe is from Chinese medicine and modern research, so aim to be asleep during those hours as much as possible.

The hour before bedtime can make or break your sleep. I used to not fully pay attention to this, even though this is what I preached every day to my patients, but after having a bout of insomnia, I no longer take this lightly.

Even if you think you sleep well, if you don't prepare for sleep properly by winding down, likely, you are not getting as much rest as you could. What's worse, your nervous system has to use your sleep as a way to relax instead of starting the healing process that happens at night. You are cheating yourself of the many benefits a lovely, deep, and prolonged sleep can do for you.

Not winding down will affect all the different types of insomniacs. The anxious type will have even more trouble falling asleep. The overthinking type will wake up at 1 a.m. full of thoughts. The overtaxed will sleep until four or five and then feel jerked out of sleep, sort of wired and feeling "on," too awake, as if on caffeine but not the good type of feeling.

Once you have established your winding down time, shift gears and intentionally slow down, devote this time to yourself and invite a sense of calm in preparation for sleep. One of the best ways to maintain that commitment is to let your family know of your plans; that way they can support and hold you accountable.

Start your winding down routine

If you are like me, proper wind down only happens if I put my devices away. Yes, some evenings, I choose to watch a movie. But most evenings, I will turn off my phone or at the least put it on airplane mode, plug in my computer, and put it away.

As a general rule, I put electronics either out of my bedroom or at least not within reach of my nightstand. Having your phone on your nightstand is too tempting. I recommend purchasing a separate clock to use as an alarm clock. Another possibility is to put your phone out of reach of your bed, so when it goes off in the morning, you get up to turn it off, so there is no lingering in bed.

When it comes to phones, tablets, and computers, I am concerned not only about the blue light emitted by electronics, which slows down melatonin production but also about the higher levels of engagement and stimulation for our brains.

Just a few weeks ago, in celebration of National Unplugging Day, I didn't use electronics for twenty-four hours at home. The twenty-four-hour period started on a Friday at 6 p.m. After eating dinner, I realized my default was watching a movie for a couple of hours. Since that wasn't a choice that night, I read a book. I started feeling incredibly groggy and sleepy about forty-five minutes in. It was way before my regular time, but that reminded me how if given a chance, your body will relax and sleep. If I had watched the movie, I would have likely been up later, would have woken up at the same time, and wouldn't have gotten the rest my body wanted.

Suppose you choose to use some electronics, and you feel quite sensitive to artificial light in the evening. In that case, I recommend blue-light-blocking glasses to help diminish the exposure to brain-stimulating light in the evenings.

After putting away your electronics, prepare your bedroom for sleep. Turn down your bed, dim your lights, and open a window for some fresh air. Then, spend the next hour doing things slowly and intently. Take time to brush your teeth and be aware of your body with each movement. Feel the muscles in your arms, legs, and shoulders. Sense the tension and stress accumulated during the day leave you little by little, moment by moment, with every task at hand.

Many of us still feel the intensity of the day buzzing in our minds, even in the evenings. The evening is a perfect time to integrate a bit of journaling into your routine—to write down your thoughts. This journaling can vary significantly in what it can contain. Whatever you choose to write can be highly beneficial in lowering your stress levels and increasing your sleep quality.

You can start this process as soon as you get home, adding more and more thoughts throughout the evening until your mind cannot think of a single ruminating thought that's not on that paper. We'll discuss this more in the following pages.

Ways to wind down before bedtime

Here are some ideas if you need guidance. You can choose one category or cover them all.

Write down your worries. Sometimes it is nice to set a timer or allocate a certain amount of time so you do not get ruminative or stuck in the worries especially if you feel anxious. It is also nice not to write the worries immediately before bed. Perhaps do it earlier before PJs and washing face.

Putting your worries down on paper will keep them from racing through your mind after the lights are out. Write down what you are worried about, and then include, "I acknowledge I am worried about this particular matter, but I choose to let go and trust that everything will work out. I will receive guidance, help, and people necessary to find a solution." Lastly, if any little steps come to mind toward easing that worry, for example, *I will call so and so tomorrow*, write it down.

Creating a list of things you must do will keep your mind clearer. It's incredible how we repeatedly go over the same thing we need to take care of in our minds. Once we write it down the first time it comes to mind, you can gently tell your mind, "Don't worry, it is written down; I got it."

Work with "I am" affirmations. Write down your desires in the "I am" form as a way of helping you to realize those dreams. For example, if I desired more financial abundance, I might write something like, "I am grateful to notice my desire, and I am noticing all the things I am abundant in already—simple things, such as plenty of water, plenty of ideas for my business or my life. I am resourceful, and I find more ways to create greater financial freedom every day. I trust, open my mind and heart to see opportunities, find the right people," and so on. Then you can add thoughts like how it would make you feel to have your desires come true—such as free, happy, creative, safe, and loved.

Make a gratitude list. If you wrote only one thing, it should be this. So much power lies in gratitude. I typically write something I am grateful for in the morning and at night. One of my friends gifted me this beautiful green jade necklace with 108 beads. It sat on my windowsill for years, and I admired it. Then one day, I heard someone saying how they use their 108 beads to say what they are grateful for—108 things to be thankful for. So, some nights, I lie in bed with the beads in my hands and start finding something I am deeply grateful for. Most nights, I fall asleep before I finish. What a beautiful way to fall asleep each night.

No matter what, do not worry about the quality of your writing or about somebody reading your thoughts. This practice is about clearing your mind for restful sleep and putting out intentions for greater happiness.

Writing about tasks and worries is particularly important for the overthinking type, as they tend to ruminate more than any other insomniac. But everyone can benefit from one form or another of journaling. Just choose what works for you and do it consistently for a few weeks before deciding whether it is helping you.

Include therapeutic touch in your evenings. Another idea for your evenings is giving and receiving touch. By sharing and accepting touch, we allow the tissue to process tension and stress and prepare us for better sleep and more inspired thoughts the next day. Touch is the first sense to develop in humans. It brings comfort and relaxation while providing a deep connection with the person you are in contact with. For this reason, some of my patients have found the firm pressure and comfort of a weighted blanket to be calming as well.

If you have a partner or a child to join in an exchange of touch, love, and relaxation, please invite them. Take turns providing at least ten minutes each. If some dedicated massage time is not viable for you, give yourself some attention and gently massage different areas of your body, focusing on your legs, shoulders, lower back, belly, arms, and even your face. You would be surprised how much tension some people hold in their bodies specifically their neck, shoulders and jaw without realizing it.

If you choose to massage your child, ask them if they would like you to rub their back or feet. Once you give them the massage, ask them if they want to reciprocate. If they do not want touch, ask how else you can help them relax without using electronics and respect their answer.

Shower to de-stress. If you typically shower at night, which I highly recommend, practice the same mindfulness of bringing awareness into your body and letting go of the stress accumulated during the day. For most people, warm water is a soothing ritual that can help relax and prepare to sleep.

Take a relaxing bath. How often do you take the time to prepare a luxurious bath for yourself? A couple of times a year? Taking a hot bath can be incredibly soothing. If that sounds attractive, take the time at least once a week or more often for a long, bubbly bath. I find bathtubs, even those home jacuzzi bathtubs uncomfortable. So my first must is to have those inflatable back pillows. They make the tub *so* much better.

Other supplies you may need are Epsom salts, essential oils, bath bombs, and whatever else pleases you. Just keep the products toxin-free. Spend twenty minutes or so soaking. Close your eyes and feel your body in the water. Observe the thoughts that go through your mind and always come back to simply feeling the water and noticing your breath. If taking a bath is impossible, shower and visualize the water taking all your worries away.

Heating your body and then stepping into a cool room tricks your body into an artificial cooling-down, which will help you feel groggier and more ready for sleep. However, for some people, taking a hot bath or shower can make them more active and anxious. In that case, either move the bath or shower earlier in the night or skip this.

Use stretching to promote relaxation. A few gentle yoga stretches in bed can feel soothing and relaxing. Start by completing all the sleep prep you've already implemented into your routine. Then, get in bed and prop yourself up with some pillows. Take a few moments to feel your body, watch your mind, and notice your breath. Once you feel in tune with your body, gently shift down and lie flat on your bed, remaining on your back. Stay there for a few moments, again, noticing your breath and feeling different parts of your body. Begin your yoga poses by hugging both knees into your chest and rocking slowly from side to side. Relax your knees, legs, and back while taking a few deep breaths. Then, continue with any of the stretches from the resource page on my website.

A relaxed mind leads to a relaxed body, and vice versa. Meditating and doing yoga can help you let go of the day's stress and worries while also allowing you to sink deeply into your bed and sleep better.

Read engaging and relaxing books. Hopefully, you now have a routine in your mind, so it's time to cap it off with some light reading. I love fiction books because they can help us escape into the story, often forgetting our worries and stresses. Reading is a great way to help you decompress and relax into the evening. But nonfiction books can also be excellent so long as they leave you feeling lighthearted.

The main goal should be to choose engaging but relaxing books. Look for those who will leave you feeling uplifted and inspired, going to bed with a smile. Then, give yourself some time at the end of your routine to read a chapter or two before shutting off the lights. If you find you can't stop reading or become overly engaged, read in a separate comfortable chair, not in bed, and limit the time.

When trying to heal from insomnia, I typically advise avoiding self-help books. As we struggle with sleep issues, reading this type of book can be triggering. The purpose is to help, but these books can sometimes bring up issues that may activate us and be counterproductive to the very goal we are reading for in the first place. Fiction books activate a more creative and less linear part of the brain. We step into someone else's shoes for a short while, and along with that, we relax.

Lastly, turn off the lights when you feel sleepy and groggy instead of just being tired, and you will have a better chance of sleeping. Feeling sleepy is particularly important if you have trouble initiating sleep.

Troubleshooting your trouble falling sleep

These are some of the scenarios that happen as people try to fall asleep.

I know I have trouble falling asleep, so I will go to sleep earlier so I have more time in bed. The problem with this is that you usually still don't fall asleep, and in fact, you may make it worse as your body is not ready for sleep. Then you start building anxiety as you lie in bed waiting.

If you notice that going to bed earlier helps with your issues, go ahead and do that. Watch how you feel at night. If you get groggy at 7 p.m. or you get a surge of energy at 9 or 10 p.m. right when you try falling asleep, taking a rest during the day may help. Read the napping section in the next chapter.

We are attempting to shift your natural highs and lows. If you take a rest or a nap around 2 p.m. even though you might not be tired then, you rest a little, hopefully delaying the low that you have at 7 p.m. to a couple of hours later, when you would like to sleep.

You're used to going to sleep at 10 p.m. because you have to wake up at six, but every night you have trouble falling asleep. It is worth trying to stay up later until you actually feel groggy and sleepy and still wake up at the same time in the morning. It might be rough for a week or two, but if you stay consistent with the wake-up time, your body will likely start learning the routine and gradually feel sleepy earlier and earlier.

Or what may happen is that you feel sleepy around 9:30 p.m. but are not ready for bed, so you rush to brush your teeth and get ready for bed, and then you are wide awake. You just had a second wind and may need another hour or two to fall asleep. If this happens to you, preparing for bed in advance is essential.

Get to know your body, and when you feel sleepy, honor that. If you get a second wind, the best course of action is not to force yourself to fall asleep. Forcing yourself to fall asleep when you are not ready doesn't work and will only cause the anxiety to build.

Know that the rush of neurotransmitters and cortisol that gave you that energy has its cycles, and you have to wait awhile. Do your best to enjoy what you do, such as reading a book; sleep will come. For some people, once they experience a rush of energy or a second wind, it is a couple of hours until they fall asleep.

Remember, we set up a desired bedtime, but it may vary a bit, depending on when we reach that sweet groggy moment. What is important is to wake up at the same time.

There are two schools of thought on this topic.

The first says to be consistent; go to sleep at the same time and wake up at the same time. The benefit is our bodies love consistency. The not-so-good part is it doesn't allow for any flexibility. What if some days I am exhausted for one reason or another? Should I not go to sleep earlier?

The second says to listen to your body, sleep when you feel sleepy, and wake up when you feel rested. I like the part about listening to our bodies; however, this may not always work, and if you don't have good boundaries, it may cause more problems. Also, we live in a society with jobs that usually require us to wake up at the same time.

My solution is a combination of the two schools of thought: Allow some flexibility in the evening, but wake up at the same time in the morning. I know I said to always aim for five or six sleep cycles—seven and a half to nine hours—but as you try to heal your insomnia while you keep those cycles in mind, you will focus less on them. After all, with choppy sleep, those cycles are likely interrupted anyway.

I like this model because it does both. It provides consistency, as your body will now learn that no matter what, you always wake at 7 a.m. Secondly, it allows you to listen to your body. You know when to go to bed, but take the pressure off and allow your body to cue you.

You can do what I do once your sleep is more solid and consistent. I typically sleep for seven and a half hours, from 10 p.m. to 5:30 or so. But some days, I am exhausted due to more physical activity than usual, more stress at work, jet lag, or an illness. In that case, I start the winding down process right after dinner and aim to fall asleep at 8:30 p.m. It can feel ridiculously early, but it's usually only one or two nights per week, if that, and then I go back to my 10 p.m. time. It works so well to recover and rest.

Life after 7 p.m.

Just when you thought, *Here it is. I got it! It's the one hour before bed that matters.* Now, I am telling you what you do after seven o'clock also matters. Seven o'clock is an approximate time when most of us are home eating dinner, done with work.

Now that you understand more about the hour before bed, is there anything you can do in the hours before that to help improve the quality of your sleep? What are you usually doing between 7 p.m. and bedtime in your typical week? Most busy professionals and parents tend to tackle their chores, and sometimes even work into the evenings. When that happens, we are frequently left feeling wired and not fully present at home.

The twelve hours of activity and twelve hours of slowing down

I like to think about our twenty-four hours split into two categories: twelve hours of activity and twelve hours of slowing down. Instead, we have about sixteen hours of activity and eight hours of passing out. There is so much more to rest than just sleeping.

In Chinese medicine, we look at the balance between yin and yang. *Yin* is about slowing down, being quieter, gently connecting with others and ourselves, and sleeping. *Yang* is activity, movement, engagement, being in the world, and social media interaction. Yin and yang are not separate but deeply interdependent. *Yin* contains a little yang, and *yang* has a little yin. So that means, throughout the day, it is good to take some time to slow down, such as a nap or simply a little rest. It also means that throughout the evening, we will do some activities that may be more yang, such as watching a movie once in a while.

In general, when these two are balanced, it is all good. If the scale is always weighted too heavily on one side, usually way too much yang and activity or doing, the balance is not there, and we gradually feel unwell.

Notice your habits and tendencies in the evening

The first step is to take the time to notice what your tendencies are in the evenings. Do you rush through chores and find yourself exhausted by the time you sleep?

Most parents, for example, would say they are making dinner, eating, putting the kids to bed, washing dishes, and then sinking into bed themselves as soon as possible.

Or are you zoning out for hours on TV or social media?

What would it look like if you found ways to make your evenings less hectic and more mindful?

How can I organize myself in the morning and during the day to be more relaxed in the evening? It is all about finding ways to work with what needs to be done to make your evenings easier and more pleasurable for you and your loved ones.

Or it may be about figuring out how not to run away from our feelings and problems, hiding away in a glass or two of wine and social media scrolling or TV watching.

Making dinner a daily relaxing routine

Dinner has the potential to be one of the best times of the day. Comforting food accompanied by our loved ones can be enjoyable, something we should all look forward to.

Unfortunately, some things might make dinnertime less exciting. For instance, preparing, cooking, and cleaning up an entire meal can dampen the whole thing, especially if you prefer to avoid cooking.

Or you may live alone and have nobody to share your dinner with.

If you live by yourself, create a routine that works for you. Preparing meals in advance always helps. Make a list of simple meal ideas for three to four days, and then come home knowing you have what you need to cook a healthy meal. Reward yourself with a dinner or lunch out a couple of times a week.

If you haven't already involved your family in helping out with dinner, now is the time. Not only will that lead to less stress in the kitchen for you, but it can also create further opportunities for bonding. Consider making an ongoing list of responsibilities for each night, with everyone taking over some aspect of cooking and cleaning. Or you may want to alternate cooking nights with your partner and/or kids so that everyone has a meal or two each week they are responsible for. Think about it. How freeing would it be to come home from work on a Thursday to dinner already waiting for you?

I encourage everyone to eat at home as much as possible. Home-cooked meals are healthier since we have more control over our chosen ingredients and their quality. I have had many patients realize they often experienced more insomnia when they ate out at certain restaurants. That was not the only reason for their insomnia, but once they started keeping track of their sleep, they noticed a definite correlation. It can be challenging to track what bothers you; it could be the additives, the type of oils, gluten contamination, even if they aimed for a gluten-free meal, and so on.

Prioritize yourself, not work

What about when we are tempted to write emails and finish work after dinner? One of the best ways to avoid this is to make a sustained effort to prioritize.

Do not simply accept that late evening is the time to do more work on your computer. Once in a while, we all have a project that may need more attention. But as a rule, try not to let your work seep into your evening routine.

Remember, *you* run your life; don't let it run you. Setting goals can bring clarity and comfort to life. But most importantly, it creates boundaries. I understand that the unpredictable is part of life. Even with that, though, organizing your life can ease the burden of unexpected events or a sleepless night. Why? Because while you are picking up the pieces of a hard day, you know in the back of your mind that this too shall pass. The challenges are temporary, and your goals can always help to get you back on track.

Create intentions and goals to create more predictability

Planning and creating goals can look very different depending on your personality. Some people thrive on making goals for each day, each week, each month, and years to come. Others are more resistant to making plans and love change and fluidity.

You can look at this as *convergent* and *divergent* personalities. If we look at the definitions of these two words, you'll see what I'm talking about.

- Convergent is about coming closer together, especially in characteristics or ideas. This type loves strategizing, clarity, and planning ahead. They thrive on making goals.
- Divergent is about finding new or different ways or develop in different directions. This type of person wants things to be open-ended, loves making changes in plans, and can thrive within those plans only as long as they can easily change them.

Some people have equal parts of both of these personality types. Regardless of which camp you fall into, there are ways to make goal-setting work for you.

Start by attempting to bring some planning into your week. Then, if you feel inclined, integrate some planning for the months and years to come. Remember that none of this has to be set in stone. But it will remind you of your dreams while also highlighting the things that overwhelm you or commitments you may want to let go of. These beginning planning stages are a great way to draw better boundaries.

Start today and write down your thoughts and observations. You may make this future goal-planning a part of your nightly journaling. Or even better, write them down earlier in the evening while your family cleans the kitchen and washes the dishes. Even for non-planners, having a list of goals can prevent those panicked 3 a.m. wake-ups. It's soothing to know your most significant ambitions and ideas for getting there have been physically committed to paper.

Once you have more clarity around your plans, goals, and boundaries, communicate with whoever needs to hear it. It may be your boss and/or your partner.

Connect with loved ones in the evening

Lastly, we are wired to connect with other people, and our relationships shape our lives. So after dinner, spend quality time with a loved one. Don't get caught up in planning something to *do*. Instead, make a point of being together, talking, and relaxing.

If you don't have a partner, think of a close friend or a family member you could make a date with. This includes yourself. In-person, by phone, or by video!

This "date" night should be about simplicity, connection, and gratitude. Sink into having a simple human-to-human connection and express gratitude for whatever you have to be grateful for, even if it's simply having that person next to you.

Good sleep is about letting go and knowing that someone has our back. That someone can be a wonderful partner, a friend, or a higher power that we may put our trust into. And go to sleep with this mantra: "I allow myself to deeply relax and know that I am protected, safe, and loved."

What to do when you wake up at night

Waking up in the middle of the night is hard. It is tough when we don't know what to do, and anxiety builds around it.

Th general advice around being awake while in bed is don't stay in bed. Get up and do something, ideally in a different room. Something like reading a book or doing a quiet activity until you feel sleepy again and then go back to bed.

This idea, along with *sleep restriction*, is widely used in the world of CBTi (cognitive behavioral therapy for insomnia). These techniques work great for some people. I encourage everyone to give it a try. To properly understand how CBTi can help you, find a qualified CBTi therapist or doctor through the American Board of Sleep Medicine or the Society of Behavioral Sleep Medicine.

Many people with chronic insomnia have deeper roots in which changing the behavior or working with relaxation techniques is not enough. Of course, I am biased, as the people who were helped by CBTi are obviously not the people I see in my clinic.

For some people, trying to stay up until 1 a.m. because all they usually sleep is five hours, hoping to get at least five consecutive hours of sleep is brutal. Perhaps their hormones are depleted, or their body and mind are stressed. Maybe they are already so sleep-deprived that this worsens their insomnia.

In some cases, after a few days of sticking with techniques such as sleep restriction, even though it's hard, some people start sleeping better. And what a relief!

For the ones where sleep won't improve, here is what worked for some of my patients. Identify what is waking you up. What wakes you up could be your bed partner moving or snoring, pets sleeping in your bed, or your pets shaking their heads with jingling neck tags. I had one patient who kept waking up at 4 a.m. to take her thyroid meds. She wanted to drink her coffee as soon as she woke up, and coffee would have had to wait if she had taken the thyroid meds when she woke up. She said she would wake up anyway, so she started taking the thyroid meds, which became a habit for her brain and body.

These little things may not be the source of your insomnia but could be making it worse, so get creative and see if small changes could help with these noises, habits, etc.

If you are awake in your bed but not anxious, lying down and resting may be beneficial; you may be getting more rest, even though you are not asleep, and you may fall back asleep faster.

If you are not anxious but have a bustling mind worrying or simply thinking a lot, reading a book or listening to a podcast may be beneficial. I like podcasts because you can set a timer on the phone, place an earbud in one ear, especially if you have a bed partner and don't want to bother them, and hopefully, you will fall asleep, and the earbud will fall out.

What you listen to can range from water sounds or music to a talk or podcast to keep your mind engaged just enough so you don't think about what makes you anxious. I like listening to a podcast because you don't need to have lights turned on, so you might have an easier time transitioning to sleep rather than reading a book and having to turn the light off and lying down.

Reading in bed is a controversial subject. We are told that only sleep and sex happens in bed, which I agree with. But if you are peacefully reading a book and staying warm, it can be easier and more comfortable than returning from another room to a cold bed and expecting to fall asleep quickly.

However, if you are awake and notice the anxiety building up and a negative relationship to the bedroom is building, I advise that you get out of bed and move to a different room to listen to something and to do activities such as reading a book or meditating.

Here are a few other techniques for falling asleep and staying sleep.

EFT (emotional freedom technique) tapping in the middle of the night is another way to get you back to sleep. Tapping can be done out loud or in silence. The idea is to relieve the stress and diminish the possible buildup of anxiety.

Meditation beads can help you focus and relax your mind; you can have necklace of beads right next to your bed. You may use them in a few different ways. The idea is to move to the next bead after an action, such as naming gratitude or a part of the body you choose to relax with each breath you take.

You might scan your body and mimic the imagery of turning off the light in your body. Attention turns lights on; as you move up the body and away, visualize turning off the light.

Humming throughout the day can be relaxing for many. Toning with different musical notes can also release tension. Alternatively, talking out loud—perhaps when nobody is around—can be freeing, rather than going in circles in our heads.

Use various apps that provide guided breathwork and meditations such as Headspace or Insight Timer. You can look up my name on Insight Timer for a sleep-inducing relaxation.

Don't use your phone in the middle of the night for more than a few moments. Using your phone is not only stimulating due to the light emitted but also too engaging to the brain. If you have a meditation bookmarked on an app, it should take only a few seconds to turn it on and put your phone down.

Healing the root cause of your insomnia is the ultimate healing; then, you don't wake up at night. But these tools and techniques can be helpful as a transition to better sleep and to use for the rest of your life when sleep is not ideal.

Summary

The hour before sleep

- Establish your ideal time and then start the winding down process an hour before.
- Prepare your bed for bedtime so you can slide into bed and fall right to sleep when sleepy.
- Choose activities that feel enjoyable and relaxing to you to encourage sleepiness.

Life after 7 p.m.

- Notice your habits in the evening and find ways to gradually ease into the evening after 7 p.m.
- Make your evening about letting go of the day and switching to the evening relaxation while spending quality time with yourself or loved ones.
- Create your intentions for the evening with activities that promote relaxation for the nervous system.

What to do when you wake up at night

- Listen to nature sounds, music, or a podcast to keep the mind focused to make it easier to fall back asleep.

- If anxiety is present, get out of bed and go to another room with a dim light on to read, meditate or do something else that helps you keep focused but relaxed.
- Use various relaxation techniques such as EFT, body scanning, or guided meditations.

CHAPTER FOURTEEN

DURING THE DAY

What you do throughout the day is often just as critical for your sleep, as the evening habits and routine.

The first hour after you wake up

The first hour of the morning may be as important as the hour before bed. The reason is that you can do a few things in the morning to shape the rest of your day.

Here are five things to include to make a difference in your sleep:

Wake up at the same time. As explained in the hour before sleep section, waking up at the same time in the morning is essential since the body relies on an inner clock and tends to be more efficient at night when it knows how much time it has left in bed.

Expose yourself to light. As soon as we wake up, a nice bright light exposure will completely shut down melatonin production and kick in other hormones that get your day going. The exposure to light can happen by walking in the neighborhood or exposing yourself for twenty minutes to a ten thousand LUX (unit of illuminance) light lamp. The light will not only help you wake up in the morning and improve your sleep at night but also improve your mood.

Eat protein for breakfast. Start your morning with a couple of cups of room-temperature or warm water. Drinking water will activate your whole body and flush your kidneys. Then, within an hour of waking up, have a hearty breakfast. Eating protein within this timeframe regulates our cortisol levels, helping us sleep better and reducing sugar cravings (University of Missouri-Columbia 2011). Combine the protein with a healthy source of carbs and fats.

Move in the morning. Exercise in the morning can also be helpful to regulate cortisol levels and encourage natural highs and lows during the day. Hence, you have a nice dip in cortisol levels and sleep peacefully at night. As little as ten minutes of movement in the morning can improve your sleep at night.

Plan your day. We are generally happier beings and more relaxed if we have some plan; jotting this down in a notebook or on your phone can work. You may also enjoy a positive psychology planner or an online project-managing platform if you have many tasks. My typical day starts with what I am grateful for, my vision for the day in just a few words, the three most important things to do that day, and random tasks that need to be done. I use the OAK positive psychology planner. You can do much more than this, but this is the basic idea that keeps me going. The idea is to avoid jumping out of bed, checking your phone, grabbing coffee, and rushing to work. Nothing about that habit is peaceful or conducive to a relaxed day. You deprive your body of a good meal, exercise, and allowing yourself to come out of sleep and peacefully start your day. What would work for you? There is always a way, even if it doesn't seem like it initially, because your life is busy.

What you do during the day

Caffeine

Let's look at your caffeine intake. How much coffee, tea, or soda are you drinking? And how late are you drinking it? You should be stopping by noon for optimal sleep, though 10 a.m. would be ideal. And remember other sources of caffeine as well. Chocolate, certain drugs, and ice cream can all be culprits. We get used to drinking caffeine, and though this might not feel like the leading cause of many people's chronic insomnia, it can be a contributor.

Caffeine consumption can confuse people who have tried to give up caffeine and still have insomnia. Until proven otherwise, I like to assume that caffeine does have something to do with insomnia. I like to either eliminate it for a few weeks or minimize it to one cup in the morning, by 10 a.m. at the latest. Since the people I see in the clinic have already tried eliminating caffeine and insomnia still exists, we know something else is preventing them from sleeping.

Once people sleep better and try to reintroduce caffeine, they realize how sensitive they are. Most people can have at least a small amount of caffeine in the morning without adverse effects that night. The half-life of caffeine, the amount of time it takes to clear one-half of the caffeine ingested, is about five hours, but according to research can vary from 1.5 to 9.5 hours (Institute of Medicine (US) Committee on Military Nutrition Research 1970). This means some of us may still be kept up late at night by the caffeine we had in the morning.

The bottom line is we try to eliminate any possible culprits since insomnia causes are multifaceted for most people, especially chronic insomnia. Then when you are well, we reintroduce them one by one.

Alcohol

Moderation and intention also applies to consumption of alcohol. Some people are highly aware that alcohol makes their insomnia worse. They try not drinking for a while but still have insomnia. Since it's not the only causative factor, they keep drinking, and alcohol consumption compounds the issue.

We take a similar approach. Stop the alcohol until sleep is better, then reintroduce different types of alcohol gradually. Drinking earlier in the evening is ideal since it will allow the alcohol to clear out of your body by the time you go to sleep.

Secondly, after your sleep is solid, we introduce one type of drink at a time and notice what happens. Some people are okay with wine but not beer while others are affected by wine but not hard alcohol. What seems to be true is that most people start having trouble from two drinks and up.

Of course, for the sake of your liver, one drink per night is wise. Also, if you choose to drink, drinking every other night or three days on and four off is what I advise. No matter how you look at it—such as wine has antioxidants—alcohol and sugar are stressful to the liver. You have to give the liver a break to take care of the many processes it is in charge of rather than focusing on detoxing alcohol each night.

If skipping alcohol a few days per week feels uncomfortable, it's time to assess your relationship with alcohol. It may be that it has become a habit. Or an addiction. Or we are simply running away from something each night. It is up to you to take a good look and figure out how to improve your relationship with alcohol to be as healthy as possible.

Exercise

Keep your evening exercise light to moderate; for instance, yin yoga, walking, or a brief bike ride. Anything more strenuous should be done earlier in the day, before 5 p.m. This will give your body time to filter through the resulting rush of hormones and neurotransmitters before settling into bed.

Generally, moderate exercise promotes good sleep while more intense exercise can cause or worsen insomnia. Trouble falling asleep with later exercise is only true for some, though. Healthy individuals with no sleep issues will have the typical, expected outcome: If you exercise hard, you sleep deep. I grew up on a farm and know this to be true from long, long work days. I would put my head on the pillow and not even move some nights.

However, exercise can sometimes worsen insomnia for the anxious type who has trouble falling asleep as well as the depleted type. In those cases, take a short break from exercise and take it easy. Allow your body to recover and rest. Most people are unaware of this: It takes energy to fall asleep and stay asleep. So if you are sleep deprived already, and you are pushing yourself hard with your exercise routine, that makes it even harder to get good rest. The body then is in a constant state of stress.

In Chinese medicine, we say "the essence" is depleted. We are born with a certain amount—for example, our genetics and our body's resilience—which typically declines as we age. We replenish this "essence" throughout our lives with good habits, good diet, exercise, nourishing sleep, and loving relationships.

We need to stop, slow down, and allow the body to focus on recovery when we are depleted. We choose to use those precious resources to heal not to spend the energy running twenty miles. I have worked with athletes on this hard choice to slow down temporarily. It's tricky because you love running, biking, or whatever it is for you, so much. You feel alive and happy while doing it and likely right afterward. Yet it is not serving you in the long term.

The good news is that the exercise break is temporary. The other good news is that stopping from something that we have been doing for a while gives us a chance to reassess how we do life. Do we love this, or do we do it out of years of habit?

Slowing down and taking a short nap—as you'll read the napping section in the next chapter—in the middle of the day can speed up the healing process. So yes, it is truly temporary, a few weeks usually, though sometimes it can be longer. Then gradually, you can start back up. One of my patients was getting ready for a triathlon, and it was not the right time for her insomnia to train for this. She desperately needed to rest for a while and stop her running and daily swimming. I talked to her about this, but this was one of the only things she felt gave her joy. Her exercise routine and training were familiar, and she did it with her friends. I decided to support her however I could with acupuncture and herbs.

A week later, she called to tell me she had fallen and sprained her ankle. The doctor had told her she needed to stop training and that the triathlon was out of the question. She felt sad and depressed for a few days, but then she grew to love her time not doing much exercise. Of course, eventually, we laughed at the situation. She had to be forced to stop with an injury to listen and give herself the much-needed healing space.

One-minute breathing to help you relax

Down-regulating the amygdala, the primal part of our brain responsible for identifying and reacting to danger, is essential to break the cycle of the continual stress we many live in. Meditation helps us do this.

If you are the busy type of person—as most of us are—and never seem to have enough time to meditate, here is an idea. Do ten one-minute meditations throughout the day. Lowered stress throughout the day is a game-changer for good sleep. We sometimes forget who we are throughout the day dictates how we sleep at night. You are still you. The stressed individual managing life during the day is the same person who sleeps at night.

Some of us need reminders to make this happen. You could stop what you are doing at the top of the hour to focus on body sensations. You can do it anywhere as long as your phone is with you and hear the reminder. If you are at your computer, stop briefly, close your eyes, and take three full breaths. Feel your body and hear the surroundings. If you are in a meeting, you can still do it. Become super aware of your environment, hear the person talking to you, look at them, and see them. You can still take three slightly deeper breaths, and likely they won't even notice. Or better, your deeper breathing will remind them to do the same.

Sit before starting the engine every time you get in the car. Take a couple of deep breaths. Stop the rush. Stop the craziness. Stop the madness. Just breathe for a few seconds. If you are late going somewhere, you need that moment of peace even more. Since you are late already, one minute won't make a difference, which may help so you won't rush in where you are going, flustered. You may bring awareness and breath when you use the restroom. Empty your mind momentarily, be aware of your body, and feel your breath. You may stop for one minute when you are about to eat. Many religions do this as a form of prayer and in thanks for the food.

Regardless of what you do in that time, be it a prayer or simply being aware of your breath, it will significantly benefit your digestion. That is important since we need nutrients to thrive and sleep well. If you can do that ten times daily, your life will gradually change. But it feels good before anything changes: your life, your sleep, and so on. It feels good right there and then when you do it. If you don't do it for future benefits, do it for yourself right now. That is what living in the present moment is. Taking who you are in that moment and being aware of where you are.

Longer meditation

If you meditate once a day, pay attention to when you most need it. Some of us wake up in the morning feeling rushed and overwhelmed. If that's the case with you, meditating in the morning may be the best time. If you have difficulty calming down in the evening, nighttime meditation could be right for you. I recommend meditating at the beginning of your winding down hour, so you can further embody and relax before you go to bed.

When you are ready to meditate, set up a timer, sit upright, and ensure you are comfortable and your back is well supported. Then, let go for fifteen minutes. The practice of meditation is not about blocking your thoughts or feelings but about staying present with the awareness of your body and your breathing while noticing and letting go of your thoughts as many times as needed! Feel your emotions or sensations without overanalyzing *why* you feel the way you do. Like this technique, I greatly enjoy the Choiceless Awareness Technique: being aware with no agenda but simply observing.

Meditation is like going to the gym. Your thoughts are the equipment. The way you practice your mind muscle is by noticing your thoughts and coming back to the present. Feel what you feel, notice your breath, and bring awareness to different areas of your body. The purpose is to stay present with whatever you are experiencing.

Sometimes it may feel like a roller coaster while others may be incredibly relaxing. Just know that wherever you are, you will benefit from this. When people tell me, "I tried to meditate, but I can't," I tell them, "But you did." It may not feel good yet. So keep going; eventually, the mind will slow down. Being gentle, kind, and physically comfortable when meditating is important since insomnia creates enough discomfort.

The sixty thousand thoughts we have every day

One of our biggest obstacles to staying in a relaxed state of mind is negative thinking. It is estimated that we have up to sixty thousand thoughts in a day; if you observe yourself, you will notice your primary inclination. Try to tally your thoughts for an hour, remaining conscious of the direction your mind wanders throughout the day. The first time you do this, you will notice something interesting; you will have many "neutral" thoughts, but upon analyzing them, you will see some hidden negative thinking. For many of us, our thinking tends toward a negative undercurrent, subtly affecting how we see the world.

Some spiritual teachings state that we have no neutral thoughts. The mind always makes a choice. If true, bringing awareness and breaking up habits will make a difference.

Simple statements such as "I shouldn't have done this or that" or habitually putting yourself down—clinging to the idea that you have a terrible memory, for instance—are doing nothing to improve your situation! That doesn't mean we should ignore what is, but finding ways to let go of a negative self-narrative can do wonders for our happiness and improve our health.

Try thinking aloud, "I am letting go of the idea that my health is always in trouble, and I am finding solutions to improve it."

Here is another simple example. A few years ago, I had these ceramic salt and pepper shakers. Unfortunately, I always grabbed the pepper and thought it was the salt. Every time I did this, I thought, *I can never remember which is which!* The thought was true enough; I never remembered. But one day, it struck me that I kept telling myself the same story, and thus the story continued to be true. So I approached the dinner table, grabbed the salt shaker—yellow, while the pepper shaker was green—and said, "Yellow is salt." It was a simple reminder, but a miracle happened; that yellow salt shaker became stuck in my head, and I haven't gotten it wrong since.

Consider writing a list of the many negative thoughts you have. Identify the nature or core of the negative thought and create a new thought pattern or story. Here is an example of someone who may be feeling insecure about something: "I let go of the belief that I am insecure and choose to see myself as confident, moving forward with every passing day. I find resources that help me heal, I find tools, I talk to the right people, and every day I see proof that I am growing more and more confident."

This practice alone can be miraculous. Sometimes we need help. We need support from a family member, friend, therapist, coach, or doctor. Whatever it is, it is all part of your healing process!

For sleep, the attempt to switch to more positive thoughts may sound like this:

- "Even though I feel like I can't ever sleep well, I let go of that thought with every passing day, or night, for that matter. I find the right people in my life to help me out. Even though I think something may be broken, something may be wrong with me, and that's why I can't sleep well. I let go of those thoughts, accept myself as I am, and know my body can heal. My body has recovered from other things in the past. I know this may be a little more stubborn, but every day my body adjusts, and I see the little good signs coming into my life. I look for helpers in the world. I open my mind since I don't know where the help will come from and in which form, but I stay firm in my belief and keep looking."

- "Even though I dwell on the anxiety of not sleeping well every day, I forgive myself. I am doing my best. I look for solutions, try new things that help me out, and find tools and techniques I resonate with, and every day gets better and better as I notice how I stick with these new habits and how they help me."
- "Even though I feel guilty and ashamed because of all these health troubles, I accept myself just as I am. I let go of this shame and guilt, I ask for help, and I can find available and affordable assistance. I see changes every day with every moment that passes. I take it step by step, but I stick to it, and I notice how, indeed, things are improving."

And so on! Make your own list, and work it. Every. Single. Day. Until your mind starts seeing another life, another narrative. And even with the ups and downs, don't give up. If it's too tiring to repeat these sorts of statements, record yourself on your phone, and then listen to them each morning.

Summary

The first hour after you wake up

- Wake up at the same time.
- Expose yourself to light, eat a breakfast that contains protein, and get some exercise.
- Plan your day so you can experience less stress and more ease throughout the day.

What you do during the day

- Monitor caffeine intake depending on your body's needs; the same with alcohol.
- Use exercise to release stress and take short moments to pause along with practicing meditation to interrupt the stress response.
- Interrupt negative thinking loops by acknowledging fears and working with these patterns to form new, more positive and constructive thinking patterns and neuropathways.

CHAPTER FIFTEEN

RELATIONSHIPS, THE POWER OF NAPS, AND YOUR SLEEP ENVIRONMENT

Your environment—both the physical environment and emotional aspects of your relationships—has a powerful impact on the quality of your sleep.

Our relationships and how they may be affecting our sleep

Part of making it through this journey called life is having a support system including wonderful friends or family—whether chosen or born with—to fall back on when things get tough. We connect with people for different reasons.

Who do you consider your friend? How much do you hang out with them? What is the quality of the time you spend together? And most importantly, how do you feel when you are around them? What about afterward?

After considering this, you can pinpoint which of your friends are a blessing. Take the time to say thank you in your heart for the gift of knowing these people. And if you feel so inclined, pick up the phone and tell those friends personally how much you appreciate them.

On the other hand, you may come to realize that some of your friends weigh you down. Maybe they don't feel good to be around or are simply toxic for you. It takes work to figure out how to navigate through such relationships. Remember one thing: if it doesn't feel good for you, it probably doesn't feel good for them, even if neither of you has consciously realized this until now.

Sometimes it takes working on your boundaries, saying no, or simply talking with your friend about what isn't working. So take the time to analyze this friendship and ask yourself if something is redeemable or if you are better off letting go. Then know it's always in your power to change the dynamics of your relationships as you gain clarity on what feels "right" for you.

What if you don't have friends or a community? There is a saying, "To make a friend, be a friend." Of course, this is easier said than done, especially for those of us who are pulled in a thousand different directions or have social anxiety. But when we find ourselves in this situation, it is always good to look at our beliefs. Deep down, do we think committing time to people we don't know is a waste? Have we been disappointed in the past? Or sometimes, is it easier to hide at home in our little cocoon?

Weigh all of this in your life and take baby steps toward trying to open up more. Make your focus simply on enjoying whatever interactions you have, and you will notice over the next year that you may make more friends.

The more intimate side of things

Do you make sure pleasure is part of your life? How is the intimacy in your relationship? And how are you nurturing yourself if you are not in a relationship?

There are many ways to invite pleasure in your life but to take the personal nature of these questions a step further: How is your sex life? Many of the people I talk to are too busy and tired even to contemplate the state of their own pleasure, but deep down, we all yearn toward feeling satisfied, more alive, and having greater intimacy.

We prioritize by putting our families, friends, jobs, or businesses first. Still, you can only take care of something to the best of your ability when you prioritize being the healthiest, happiest version of yourself. You owe it to yourself to take care of yourself and notice your personal needs—sexual and otherwise.

As women, fluctuating hormones and stages of a cycle are an opportunity to slow down, shift our focus, and take care of ourselves. That may mean resting more, reading more, or watching a movie on your own—whatever feels nurturing to you. Communication with your partner is another way to bring awareness to your normal fluctuating hormones, bringing understanding and greater intimacy.

Having intercourse in the evening before going to sleep can be too activating for some people. If that is the case, communicate your needs with your partner. This communication is essential since, often, between family, job, and kids, you may never feel like it's the right time for pleasure and physical expression of love with your partner.

In addition, look at your ability to express your desires, fears, and worries. Talking about your sexuality and intimacy can be challenging, but the rewards are beautiful and can bring you closer to your partner or help you find one.

To be more practical, take action and take care of your health if your hormones and neurotransmitters are imbalanced. Hormonal imbalances are prevalent in sleep issues, and this can affect your mood, libido, energy levels, and sleep quality.

Napping to help heal your insomnia

Our bodies are biologically optimized to take a siesta in the afternoon. Naps are not popular in our culture, but they can help us in many ways. Naps can be seen as lazy, something that only babies do, or that something is wrong with you if you need a nap. So there is a bit of negative talk around this subject, but I see it as rebooting and recharging our internal computer.

Napping has multiple benefits. We have a natural dip in body core temperature and a minor release of melatonin in the early afternoon, so we are made for afternoon naps. We have a more significant core temperature dip at night, which helps us feel groggy before bedtime.

Each twenty-four hours acts like a wave with highs and lows. We have a tremendous upward wave in the morning to get our day going, a slight dip in the afternoon, another upward surge late in the afternoon, and a more significant drop to prepare to ease into sleep. When we take a nap, we strengthen that healthy curve, we increase our energy in the afternoon; and we will likely sleep better at night.

Dozing, even for just a few minutes can feel refreshing. You feel better, and your mood is improved. You feel ready to take on the rest of the day easily. We interrupt the stress response when we nap. Every time I lie down in bed to take a quick nap, I take a deeper breath a few minutes in, which tells me I have been holding my breath. That moment of relaxation is one of the most important things you can do for your body to heal and prevent disease.

As an additional benefit, research shows that midday napping is associated with lower blood pressure (American College of Cardiology 2019).

We also typically find ourselves more alert, productive, and happy after a nap. Truthfully, it just feels so darn good. That's why I do it! Nothing else will make my afternoon better in every way possible.

Before we discuss how to nap, let me tell you about the three types of napping to consider.

1. **Planned napping:** when you know you will have an extra-demanding afternoon/evening or plan to be out late at night.
2. **Habitual napping:** daily, almost daily, or weekend napping. For example, I nap once or twice a week as my schedule allows and almost always on Saturdays and Sundays.
3. **Emergency napping:** the absolute minimum that you could give yourself if the other two are not feasible for you. It would be best to have an emergency nap when not doing so might be dangerous for you or others, like if you're driving a car and feeling sleepy. For your sake

and that of others, you must pull over, recline your seat, and take a little nap. Do not think, *I will be all right.* You need to stop what you're doing and find a way to rest.

There are two different schools of thought when it comes to napping. The first believe you shouldn't ever nap, especially if you have insomnia. The second say napping is good for you. I recommend napping often, especially for people who suffer from the anxious or depleted type of insomnia, though most types and people can benefit.

Here's how to nap to help you feel less stressed and less tired in order to improve your sleep at night:

- Your napping period has to end about seven or eight hours before bedtime. For example, if your bedtime is ten, nap from 1 to 3 p.m. If you fall asleep closer to midnight or even after midnight and wish to move your clock and be able to fall asleep earlier, I still recommend napping no later than 3 p.m. This timeframe encourages the healthy cycle of a natural dip around 2 p.m. followed by an increase in energy and a natural drop earlier in the night instead of closer to midnight.
- Keep the nap short. Unless you are sick or sleep-deprived from traveling, in which case a ninety-minute nap may be acceptable, keep your naps under thirty minutes. If they go longer than that, you will wake up groggy rather than rested.
- Set the alarm for thirty minutes, so you can just let go and relax. Do so even if you tend to wake up on your own before that time. Then you can enjoy those moments instead of worrying that you might oversleep. If you can't nap, lying down for thirty minutes can be helpful.

Eventually, if you do it often enough, you might start dozing off. Lying down still encourages that natural dip and is soothing to the nervous system.

- Make it cozy and sweet. I tend to climb into my bed, under the covers, put my sleep mask on, and enjoy that beautiful moment of quiet. If your mind keeps racing, listening to a meditation may be helpful. Get creative if you can't make it to your bed for a nap. Some of my patients have napped in their cars. They brought a blanket and pillow or a sleeping bag and pillow to their office, closed their door, and drifted off to dreamland. If you have later afternoon dips in energy, always try to nap right before it happens. I say this because my patients often complain that they get tired and want to sleep around 3 or 4 p.m. when it's too late to nap. Catch it before it happens.

If you have insomnia and feel like the more exhausted you are, the harder it is to sleep, focus on napping. This is the type of insomnia that best improves with napping.

These are some ideas on how to make napping work for you. Try a handful of times before deciding whether it's working for you.

If fatigue affects your life, there may be other medical reasons why you are so tired rather than being sleep-deprived.

About your sleep environment

You want your bedroom to be a relaxing and soothing place. It should be clean, organized, and decorated with colors that soothe you. Our bedroom is where we spend one-third of our lives, and while we are not awake to observe it, it still matters. If our bedroom is cluttered, we tell ourselves to a certain degree that this space is unimportant. If you live in clutter and your bedroom is not the only place like that, it's time to start somewhere; it might as well be the bedroom!

Shop for natural-fiber sheets, such as cotton. The type of fibers is critical if you experience hot flashes and/or night sweats since synthetic fibers trap the heat.

A dark bedroom is crucial for better sleep because the pineal gland, which produces melatonin, is stimulated by darkness and inhibited by light. Use blackout blinds or curtains and consider a silk sleep mask. I like the room so dark I can't see my palm after lying in bed for a few minutes when I lift my hand up. It will help you sleep more deeply and wake up less.

When we complete one sleep cycle, which lasts about ninety minutes, we enter the second sleep cycle. Any stimulants, such as a small amount of light, might pull us out of sleep. The melatonin production will be enhanced the darker our sleep environment is.

Avoid charging your phone or using a radio-type alarm clock on your nightstand. Not charging near your bed decreases the electric field emitted next to your head. As far as electromagnetic fields, I also recommend turning off the Wi-Fi at night. You can put your Wi-Fi on a timer, found at any hardware store—and set it to automatically turn off around 10 or 11 p.m. Then turn it back on in the morning at your desired time.

Clean air in your bedroom is important since we spend so much time in it. An air purifier is best, but if you don't have allergies and live in a clean area, opening the windows can also help. Look for air purifiers with various filters, such as HEPA and carbon.

Sleeping with a bed partner who moves a lot, snores, or has a CPAP machine on can also be pretty disturbing for your sleep. I often recommend sleeping in different beds, at least temporarily, until the insomnia gets better. We live in a society where sleeping in separate beds is stigmatized, but a discussion between partners usually helps soften this up. The advantage of this is that it may benefit intimacy since it's a partner's intentional choice to visit each other.

The temperature in the bedroom is also critical. We sleep better at cooler temperatures as long as our bodies, especially hands and feet, are warm. According to The Sleep Foundation, sixty to sixty-eight degrees Fahrenheit is ideal for sleep for most individuals (Pacheco and Wright 2023).

I also suggest reviewing the toxic burden chapter for more things you can do in your bedroom to improve your sleep.

Summary

Our relationships:

- Focus on relationships that nourish you and bring you happiness.
- Work on creating boundaries with "friends" that leave you drained and uninspired.
- Invest time in building a supportive community if that is what you desire.

The more intimate side of things:

- Take some time to ponder how pleasure is present in your life and how you can invite more of it.
- Communicate with your partner about your desires and needs to bring more fulfillment.
- Balance reproductive hormones and neurotransmitters.

Napping to help your insomnia:

- Find time to nap as a way to relax the nervous system, either every day or as needed.
- Nap seven hours or more before your bedtime. Set up a timer for thirty minutes and focus on resting.

About your sleep environment:

- Keep your bedroom free of clutter and chemicals and use natural fibers on your bed.
- The darker the bedroom the easier is to fall asleep and stay asleep.
- Keep the temperature sixty to sixty-eight degrees Fahrenheit.

PART V

SUMMARY

Congratulations for making it here and reading these words. This final chapter is here for you to help you design your healing protocol by reviewing the insomniac types along with next steps for sleep healing.

CHAPTER SIXTEEN

TYING IT ALL TOGETHER AND STARTING TO CREATE YOUR HEALING PROTOCOL

Before we review the insomniac types, here are some action steps to guide you if you haven't already started implementing a healing protocol:

- Identify which type of insomniac you are and which healing chapter may apply.
- Look into the stress response system and see what changes you can make.
- Identify the best sleep hygiene steps for you.
- Go deep into the primary system affected, besides the stress response, and work on healing it.
- If you need help figuring out where to start, begin with the gut and the elimination diet.
- Look for a practitioner to help you further.

Let's review the insomniac types and how they relate to the healing sections.

The anxious insomniac

A sense of anxiety is at the forefront of most insomniacs. However, suppose you identify yourself with the anxious insomnia type. In that case, no matter the root cause, focusing on the tools and practices that help soothe your nervous system is crucial.

Review the stress response chapter and then refer to sleep foundations chapter. Choose what you resonate with the most, and start implementing it in your life. You will need a few weeks of learning about yourself, what works for you, and what doesn't.

Two things to remember: Anything you try, give it a fair try, not just once or twice. An honest attempt may mean one to three weeks or even longer, depending on the situation. Be patient. Changing habits and sleep patterns take time. Second, some things will feel miraculous; others take consistency to make a difference. You want to focus on more than the end product but rather how it feels in the moment.

When I drink my golden milk tea with ashwagandha in the morning or evening, I don't ask myself after a few days, *Do I feel less stressed?* What I say is, *Does it feel and taste good?* Yes, it's warm, tasty, nourishing, and delicious. Some people who start napping, or resting for thirty minutes in the afternoon don't doze off for a few weeks or sometimes never. The aim is to rest, so how does it feel? Can you relax by lying down, feeling warm, listening to something pleasant, letting your mind go, being relaxed, and permitting yourself to do nothing for those thirty minutes? The body and mind will eventually get the message to let go in the middle of the day.

For women, I often see how their insomnia can be related to hormone imbalances on top of nervous system dysregulation.

For men, when this pattern is present, especially with early awakenings, I recommend screening for sleep apnea.

For both, looking at possible chronic infections is also wise and sometimes the root cause of why the nervous system is so on edge and these people cannot sleep well. In addition, for most insomniacs but especially the anxious type, it is recommended to test for pyroluria.

The overthinking insomniac

A tendency to process and ruminate is present in this pattern. The sleep foundations chapters will be helpful to you. It was likely obvious to you while reading what steps could be beneficial. If not, revisit that chapter and see what would help put your mind at ease. As mentioned in the previous type, allow time to create new patterns, and focus on how it feels while you do it, not so much grasping at the result. If you think and worry about the change you decided to make, about whether this particular change will have the outcome you desire, that defeats the purpose of your healing as the overthinking insomniac type. So you must live in the moment and pick things you enjoy doing to stay in the present moment.

Your best bet to go back to sleep is not trying—especially not trying hard. This applies to all the insomniac types. There is a saying: "What do good sleepers do to fall asleep?

Nothing." Of course, the answer is not as simple as that, but in those moments when you lie down in bed intending to sleep, there should ideally be no forcing, no striving, no wondering. You are just there, enjoying the bed, letting some fleeting thoughts come and go, and the next thing you know it's the morning.

Since you are struggling with insomnia, this concept of just doing nothing, as simple as it is, sounds maddening. You may do nothing for ten or even thirty minutes, and if you are not asleep, you can't help but start worrying about all sorts of things. The aim is to heal the root cause of why you can't sleep, but as a transition, we have to gradually teach the body and mind to become confident again. Go back to the sleep foundations chapters and comb through it. What would be helpful for you? Would starting to jot things down around 5 or 6 p.m., until your mind is empty, be beneficial? Is having many choices of music, bedtime stories, guided meditations, or podcasts all lined up on your phone, ready to go, helpful when you can't fall asleep?

Then assess your digestion. At the very least, go through an elimination diet for four weeks. That may require the support of a healthcare provider who understands this diet so you can make sure you do your best with it.

For women, when waking up in the middle of the night, typically around 1 or 2 a.m., there is often a hormonal imbalance component. Sometimes it is obvious, such as when waking up because of a hot flash or night sweat; at other times, it is not but could still be related to hormonal imbalances, so work with a practitioner for further support.

The overtaxed insomniac

If I had to choose a type that is the epitome of our busy society, this would be it. But I can tell you the anxious and overthinking type are right there, trailing close behind. This type is more directly related to our perpetual stress while the first two can be a little more complex in roots and causes.

Since the most common pattern for this type is waking up early in the morning, sometimes it is not evident that the insomnia may be due to unprocessed stress. The connection can feel more pronounced when we can't fall asleep because we are anxious or worried.

The way I look at it is this: You are exhausted, so you, thankfully, fall asleep, but after some necessary four or five, or even six hours of sleep, your body and mind say, "Oh, that's plenty for survival. Let's get up to be on the watch for the danger." Of course, the danger is not the wild animal, but it hasn't been long since we were cavemen and women, so the instincts are alive. It doesn't matter if we worry about a problem to be solved at work or have anxiety about a conversation we must have with a loved one. The same stress response is active.

This type often has a cortisol rise too early in the morning. As time passes, the natural cortisol curve throughout the day and night changes, and we may start getting sleepy in the afternoon, only to have too much energy in the evening, and then we cannot fall asleep at our usual time.

It may seem counterintuitive, but working on the winding down process in the evening is crucial for early morning insomnia. Also, how you deal with waking up early is essential. If it's way too early, ninety minutes or more before it is time to get up, it is best to stay in bed as long as you can do so peacefully. Having a variety of resources and tools easily accessible to listen to or read can be helpful. Since it's hard to fall back asleep, this is nurture time. In these moments, I try to let go of the fact that I would rather be sleeping deeply and see it as "extra" time that I wouldn't have had otherwise. So I use it to listen to books or guided meditations that take an hour or longer. Do the thing that is relaxing, and you otherwise wouldn't have the time for during the day. This time of relaxation can often lead to some dozing off.

It's tempting to sleep in when we wake up too early and then doze off, but it is best to stick with a consistent getting out of bed time to create a routine for your body. I don't encourage people to get up when waking up too early to help the body understand it is meant to sleep until your desired time. But if you sleep in some of the mornings past that time, it defeats the purpose of the first goal and confuses the body.

The overtaxed insomnia type can be due to emotional and mental stress. Still, this type can spill into all the other categories, and the root cause can range from digestive issues to hormonal imbalances, toxic burden, liver issues, chronic infection, pyroluria, or sleep apnea.

The depleted insomniac

If you have resonated with this or the following type, you will read this book and want to tell everyone about it. Because finally, you now understand why your insomnia wasn't just in your head and why it wasn't as simple as taking an herb or medication to heal! You may feel like, *"Finally, I understand what I already knew; something complex is going on that causes me not to sleep well."*

Any of the chapters contained in this book may be relevant to you. Though primarily, you may have found yourself in one or two and are now willing to take the steps discussed. It will take some patience, so it is best to have professional support to make real progress, especially if you need to get clarity on what to start with.

Testing may be necessary to grasp why you haven't been able to sleep for a long time, as each depleted insomniac type will usually have had trouble sleeping for many years.

Before digging deeper into root causes, I often recommend testing cortisol and neurotransmitter levels to use those as a jumpstart, at least for symptom relief. Then, based on your other symptoms, look at the different systems where the main imbalances may be found.

"When in doubt, start with the gut" is a common saying in the holistic medical community. You can't go wrong with maximizing digestion and balancing the gut microbiome. Especially because of the gut-brain axis connection!

Above all, give yourself space and rest as much as possible. I call it "the depleted" type for a reason. Don't get me wrong. Many of you in this category are perfectly capable of doing life; however, to heal, you need to slow down, be gentle, and allow time for the process. If you have insomnia, you need a certain degree of rest and gentleness. We can create no better foundation for ourselves to safely and completely let go at night.

The overburdened insomniac

One of the primary descriptions of this type is feeling like something is irritating your system. Other than that, it may feel like the overthinking type, anxious type, or even the overtaxed type. Sometimes people will say something like, "It's like something pulls me out of sleep," "Something doesn't let me sleep," or "I feel like I am being poisoned." Some of us may not be as aware, but if you resonate strongly with this type and you need help knowing where to start, you should reach out to a healthcare professional.

Another place to start is to look around your environment and, based on what you read here, see what makes the most sense to change. Eliminating sources of toxicity may have an immediate effect, but that is not always true.

Is your body capable of detoxing what it has accumulated and retained for months or years? The next step would be to start a gentle detoxification protocol. The most impactful way to start is with food. The modified elimination diet in the toxic burden chapter offers guidance to get you started. Do not underestimate the power of consistently feeding your body lots of vegetables and good quality protein, fats, and carbs over a few months. You will look back and pleasantly notice the changes. The trick is to learn how to gradually let go of what is not beneficial in your body while at the same time feeding your body nutritious foods. This applies to sleep foundation changes, too.

These are some guiding questions. What could be overburdening you? What could be toxic in your relationships? Remember that when we try to let go of something toxic, whether emotional or physical, the body's balance will be disturbed. It must learn how to adjust to achieve a new type of balance.

Change is not easy because the transition is uncomfortable. That is why we all secretly hope for instant healing, but we are not ready if you think about it. Most of us are only prepared for a gradual healing process, so we can adjust and feel at least some safety.

In Closing

We are created to live in balance, which is an active state where the body intuitively makes adjustments at all times. I know each human being is capable of incredible healing. With this being said, I wish you great healing and sweet dreams!

ACKNOWLEDGMENTS

First and foremost, I want to thank my patients who have given me the valuable gift of allowing me to practice this medicine. I am grateful for their patience with my always-evolving practice. Because of them I was able to write this book.

To King, my beloved Labrador, who is now in spirit but has quietly sat beside me through writing the first draft of this book. His presence offered me comfort and strength when I got too tired or didn't trust I could follow through and keep writing.

Thank you to Melissa. There are not enough words to express my gratitude for her help. She has not only read the manuscript and offered mindful and valuable feedback, but she has offered countless words of encouragement, at all times of the day and night over the past few years. She has reminded me to keep going in some of my darkest moments and celebrate the many wins. This book would not be where it is today if not for her. I am forever grateful.

Thank you to Victoria, my mom; in every new project, every new step, thank you for always being excited for me and praying for me. And to my whole family, for their steady prayers that this book comes to print.

Thank you to Rory for helping me keep focused when overwhelm and distractions would have me wanting to do anything else but edit my book. His steady support got me back on task many times so you can have this book in your hands today.

Thank you to Carmen, Merrill, and Melinda for some great laughter, gentle pushes, and for hugging me when tears flowed, when everything felt a bit too hard.

Thank you to Carol for helping me brainstorm and move this book along, especially its title.

Thank you to my coach and therapists, Dawn, Leanne, and Julie. They have helped sort myself through the ups and downs of life; their counsel not only kept me sane but helped me thrive and enjoy being alive.

I want to give thanks to Timothy for being there when I had the first thought to specialize in sleep disorders, and encouraging this path for many years after.

Thank you to Dr. Hamid Montakab for his unique work in Acupuncture and Chinese medicine and sleep disorders. His books and seminars inspired my sleep-focused clinical practice. I am deeply grateful to him.

Thank you to my editor Heather for the continuous support and her help in pacing myself every time I panicked. Her support felt deeper than I expected to come from an editor, it gave me comfort and confidence that I could follow through with this wild editing journey.

To all the beta readers in the past three-plus years. Thank you to Dr. Johnson and Dr. Lutz for making time in their busy schedule and offering feedback when I needed it the most. I also want to thank Dr. Timiras for her honest feedback and powerful guidance. Thank you to Dr. Jill and Dr. Wentz for their assistance. And thank you to all the first beta readers, Dr. Parrish, Dr. Hamid, Mary, Traci, Zac, Luminita, Alison, Sue, Lauren, Brodie, Erika, and Daniel.

Thank you to the Manuscripts LLC team: Heather, Angela, Venus, Eric, Stephanie, Amanda, Noemi, Gjorgji, Zvonimir, and the many people who made this book happen. I appreciate all of the support you have provided to publish my book and make this dream come true.

And a massive thank you to everyone who preordered *The Deep Blue Sleep* during the presale campaign and made the publishing of this book possible. I have been brought to tears in gratitude for the support and trust I've received. Thank you from the bottom of my heart to all of you. I couldn't have done this without you. Names are listed in alphabetical order.

Camelia Ades*
Veronica Alexeev
Ekaterina Anderson
Taylor Anderson
Jenny Bader Lyn
Cosmina Barbat
Nichole Barnett
Erin Bauman

Anne Beach
Sue Bee*
Kimberly Benjamin
Tearson Bickmore
Helen Biggar
Pamela Boll*
Megan Bullock
Carmen Burke*
Pam Burns*
Dean Campbell
Rebeca Castella*
Amanda Cattaneo
Callie Cavanaugh
Bonnie Ceres
Ira Chaleff
Karen Chiabotti*
Lee Coburn
Corinne Conry
Rory Cooper*
Barry Cooper*
Maria Cooper
Sandy Cooper*
Frances Cottingham-Kelly*
Leslie Coy*
Paula Crandall
Kathleen Crane*
Nathalie Dahouas
Louise Davis
Diane Dimeff
Ralitsa Dimitrova*
Wendy Dinkins
Michelle Dodd
Anita Dolliver
Roxana Dondera
Chris Doran
Eric Dorninger*
Marion Down
Jessica Doyle
Carmen Dragan
Seth Drake
Molly Dyer
Monica Edlauer
Elise Edson
Bob Egeland
Gabriela Enache
Marije Adinda Fagerström
Emily Fickett
Jake Fratkin
Gwendolyn Fuehring
Kym Garrett
Trevor Gauthier*
Hanna Gissler
Luminita Gogan
Nancy Goodman
Nancy Grady*
Karli Gronholm
Tamara Haisfield
Brent Hartman
Becca Haydon
Karen Hershman
Rose Honor
Michael Huttner
Chris Janeczko
Carol Johnson

Jennifer Johnson*
Florence Jones*
Merrill Jones-Barradale*
Lauren Jordan
John Joseph
Angela Justis
Steve Justus
Karen Kaufman*
Valerie Kindred
Cheri King
Eric Koester
Jeff Kraft
Angie Krause
Holly Lange
Landon Latoski
Razvan Lazarescu
Sally Lewien*
Sheila Liewald
Heather Lind
Matthew Lish*
Brandon Lockhart
Gillian Longley
Lisa Lourey*
Kevin Lutz
Anna Teresa Mahaffy*
Jesse Markt
Cinthia Martell
Betsey Martens
Leanne Massi
Abby Matsumoto
Debbie McCarthy*
Linda McCoy
Jill McIntyre
Katrina McLaughlin
Melinda McClelland*
Joe Medrano*
Carmen Merten*
Kareen Milard
Andrew Miles
Jean Murphy
Susannah Neal
Miriam Ofek Emuna
Dr. Rosia Parrish*
Debbie Patnaude
Marenca Patrascoiu
Katie Pegg
George Petredean*
Georgiana Prodan
Jazmine Quinn
Francesca Quinn*
Dianna Rands
Nick Redding
Jane Reynolds*
Carolyn Richards
John Rinaldi
James Ripley
Wyman Robb
Alex Roetter
Max Rosenshein
Rita Rosson
Stefanie Rothert
Barry Rubin*
Colleen Ryan
Kate Salama

Melisa Sanzone
Mark Saunders
Laura Scarpa-Regnere
Robin Schaefer
Gabriela Scharf
Anca Sisu
Ralf Socher
Allison Soffer
Laura Spurlock
Debbie Steinbock
Jill Stiller
Sabine Stix
Michael Stone
Linda Strader*
Farah Sultan
Karina Tibble Maria
Dawn Todd*
Cornelia Toderica
Ann Trione Marie
Stephanie Trzaska
Danijela Tunjic
David Tusek*
Courtney Walsh*
Taber Ward
Kathy Wellman
Michael Wentz
Melanie West*
Andrew Whitelaw
Rawls Whittlesey
Gerry Wienholt
Leandra Wills
Susan Wiser
Melissa Wolak
Jenna Wolf*
Barbara Woltz
Dorothy Yewer
Meredith Young
Kelly Zamecki
Brittany Zimmerman*
Nancy Van Loon

* multiple copies purchased

Many people have helped me along this book journey. Even if your name is not written here, please know it is written on my heart and your aid was not forgotten.

APPENDIX

Chapter 2

Mayo Clinical Staff. 2023 "Sleep Apnea." *Mayo Foundation for Medical Education and Research* (blog). April 6, 2023. https://www.mayoclinic.org/diseases-conditions/sleep-apnea/symptoms-causes/syc-20377631.

Richardson, Michael W. 2019. "How Much Energy Does the Brain Use?" *BrainFacts.org* (blog). February 1, 2019. https://www.brainfacts.org/brain-anatomy-and-function/anatomy/2019/how-much-energy-does-the-brain-use-020119.

Chapter 3

Cacho, Valerie, and Esther Lum. 2021. *Integrative Sleep Medicine (Weil Integrative Medicine Library).* New York: Oxford University Press.

Terry, Natalie, and Kara Gross Margolis. 2017." *Gastrointestinal Pharmacology.* 319-342. Switzerland: Springer Nature.

Chapter 4

Hirotsu, Camila, Sergio Tufik, and Monica Levy Andersen. 2015. "Interactions Between Sleep, Stress, and Metabolism: From Physiological to Pathological Conditions." *Sleep Science* 8, no. 3: 143-152. https://doi.org/10.1016/j.slsci.2015.09.002.

Chapter 5

Michaud, Mark. 2013. "To Sleep, Perchance to Clean." *News* (blog), University of Rochester Medical Center. October 17, 2013. https://www.urmc.rochester.edu/news/story/to-sleep-perchance-to-clean.

Chapter 6

Liu, Yun-Zi, Yun-Xia Wang, and Chun-Lei Jiang. 2017. "Inflammation: The Common Pathway of Stress-Related Diseases." *Frontiers in Human Neuroscience*, 11: 316. https://doi.org/10.3389/fnhum.2017.00316.

Chapter 7

Amen, Daniel. 2013. "The Most Important Lesson from 83,000 Brain Scans | Daniel Amen | TEDxOrangeCoast." TEDx Talks. October 16, 2013. 14:36. https://youtu.be/esPRsT-lmw8.

Everly, George S., Jeffrey M. Lating, and Melvin A. Gravitz. 2019. *A Clinical Guide to the Treatment of the Human Stress Response*. New York, NY: Springer.

Selye, Hans. 1976. *Stress in Health and Disease*. Stoneham, MA: Butterworths.

The American Institute of Stress. 2011. "America's #1 Health Problem." *The American Institute of Stress* (blog). October 19, 2011. https://www.stress.org/americas-1-health-problem.

Weiss, Howard D., and Laura Marsh. 2012. "Impulse Control Disorders and Compulsive Behaviors Associated with Dopaminergic Therapies in Parkinson Disease." *Neurology. Clinical Practice* 2, no. 4: 267-274. https://doi.org/10.1212/CPJ.0b013e318278be9b.

Chapter 8

Cheng, Li-Hao, Yen-Wenn Liu, Chien-Chen Wu, Sabrina Wang, and Ying-Chieh Tsai. 2019. "Psychobiotics in Mental Health, Neurodegenerative and Neurodevelopmental Disorders." *Journal of Food and Drug Analysis* 27, no. 3: 632-648. https://doi.org/10.1016/j.jfda.2019.01.002.

Dalton-Smith, Saundra. 2019. *Sacred Rest: Recover Your Life, Renew Your Energy, Restore Your Sanity*. Read by Saundra Dalton-Smith. New York: Faith Words. Audible. 7h 15min.

Feng, Yu, Xin-Yu Wang, Shao-Dan Li, Yin Zhang, Hai-Ming Wang, Min Li, Ke Cao, Yu-Fei Ye, and Zhao Zhang. 2011. "Clinical Research of Acupuncture on Malignant Tumor Patients for Improving Depression and Sleep Quality." *Journal of Traditional Chinese Medicine* 31, no. 3: 199-202. https://doi.org/10.1016/s0254-6272(11)60042-3.

Hanaway, Patrick. 2022. "Gastrointestinal Dysfunction, Chronic Disease, and the Functional Medicine Matrix Model." The Institute for Functional Medicine GI Advanced Practice Module 2022 Conference Recordings, Restoring Gastrointestinal Equilibrium: Practical Applications for Understanding,

Assessing, and Treating Gut Dysfunction. Livestream. October 2, 2022.

Kim, Young-Dae, In Heo, Byung-Cheul Shin, Cindy Crawford, Hyung-Won Kang, and Jung-Hwa Lim. 2013. "Acupuncture for Posttraumatic Stress Disorder: A Systematic Review of Randomized Controlled Trials and Prospective Clinical Trials." *Evidence-Based Complementary and Alternative Medicine* 2013: 1-13. https://doi.org/10.1155/2013/615857.

Luo, Wen-Zheng Qing-Zhong Zhang, Xin-Sheng Lai. 2010. "[Effect of Acupuncture Treatment of Relieving Depression and Regulating Mind on Insomnia Accompanied with Depressive Disorders]." *Zhongguo Zhen Jiu* 30, no. 11: 899-903. https://pubmed.ncbi.nlm.nih.gov/21246844/.

Natural Medicines Comprehensive Database Consumer Version. 2022. "Ashwagandha." *MedlinePlus*. Accessed August 2, 2022. https://medlineplus.gov/druginfo/natural/953.html.

Shekarchi, Maryam, Homa Hajimehdipoor, Soodabeh Saeidnia, Ahmad Reza Gohari, and Morteza Pirali Hamedani. 2012. "Comparative Study of Rosmarinic Acid Content in Some Plants of Labiatae Family." *Pharmacognosy Magazine* 8, no. 29: 37-41. https://doi.org/10.4103/0973-1296.93316.

Sjöstedt, Peter, Jesper Enander, and Josef Isung. 2021. "Serotonin Reuptake Inhibitors and the Gut Microbiome: Significance of the Gut Microbiome in Relation to Mechanism of Action, Treatment Response, Side Effects, and Tachyphylaxis." *Frontiers in Psychiatry* 12: 1-7. https://doi.org/10.3389/fpsyt.2021.682868.

Spence, D Warren, Leonid Kayumov, Adam Chen, Alan Lowe, Umesh Jain, Martin A Katzman, Jianhua Shen, Boris Perelman, and Colin M Shapiro. 2004. "Acupuncture Increases Nocturnal Melatonin Secretion and Reduces Insomnia and Anxiety: A Preliminary Report." *The Journal of Neuropsychiatry and*

Clinical Neurosciences 16, no. 1: 19-28. https://doi.org/10.1176/jnp.16.1.19.

Tu, Jung-Hung Wei-Ching Chung, Chun-Yuh Yang, Dong-Sheng Tzeng. 2012. "A Comparison between Acupuncture Versus Zolpidem in the Treatment of Primary Insomnia." *Asian Journal of Psychiatry* 5, no. 3: 231-235. https://doi.org/10.1016/j.ajp.2011.12.003.

Yan, Xing-ke, Yan Zhang, Lu Yu, Gong-lei Yue, Tie Li, Cheng Chen, Hai-fu Cui, and Fu-chun Wang. 2010. "[Effect on Tranquilizing and Allaying Excitement Needling Method on Brain Blood Flow in the Patients of Insomnia of Heart and Spleen Deficiency]." *Zhongguo Zhen Jiu* 30, no. 2: 113-116. https://pubmed.ncbi.nlm.nih.gov/20214067/

Zhou, Yan-Li, Xi-Yan Gao, Pei-Yu Wang, and Shan Ren. 2012. "Effect of Acupuncture at Different Acupoints on Expression of Hypothalamic GABA and GABA(A) Receptor Proteins in Insomnia Rats." *Zhen Ci Yan Jiu* 37, no. 4: 302-307. http://www.ncbi.nlm.nih.gov/pubmed/23140052.

Chapter 9

Acbay, Ozer, Aykut Ferhat Celik, Pinar Kadioglu, Suha Goksel, and Sadi Gundogdu. 1999. "Helicobacter Pylori-Induced Gastritis May Contribute to Occurrence of Postprandial Symptomatic Hypoglycemia." *Digestive Diseases and Sciences* 44: 1837-1842. https://doi.org/10.1023/A:1018842606388.

Fang, Jiliang, Danhong Wang, Qing Zhao, Yang Hong, Yulian Jin, Zhishun Liu, Kehua Zhou, Xianghong Jing, Xiaochun Yu, Ruiqi Pan, Andrew Chang, Hesheng Liu, and Bing Zhu. 2015. "Brain-Gut Axis Modulation of Acupuncture in Functional Dyspepsia: A Preliminary Resting-State fcMRI Study." *Evi-*

dence-Based Complementary and Alternative Medicine 2015: 1-11. https://doi.org/10.1155/2015/860463.

Faries, Peter L., Ronald J. Simon, Arthur T. Martella, Martin J. Lee, and George W. Machiedo. 1998. "Intestinal Permeability Correlates with Severity of Injury in Trauma Patients." *The Journal of Trauma: Injury, Infection, and Critical Care* 44, no. 6: 1031-1036. https://doi.org/10.1097/00005373-199806000-00016.

Fasano, Alessio. 2020. "All Disease Begins in the (Leaky) Gut: Role of Zonulin-Mediated Gut Permeability in the Pathogenesis of Some Chronic Inflammatory Diseases." *F1000Research* 9: 1-13. https://doi.org/10.12688/f1000research.20510.1.

Gardner, Christopher D., Justin Sonnenburg, and Scarlett Karakash. 2023. *Maternal & Offspring Microbiome Study (MOMS)*. Stanford, CA: Stanford University.

Hakim, Fahed, Yang Wang, Alba Carreras, Camila Hirotsu, Jing Zhang, Eduard Peris, and David Gozal. 2015. "Chronic Sleep Fragmentation During the Sleep Period Induces Hypothalamic Endoplasmic Reticulum Stress and PTP1b-Mediated Leptin Resistance in Male Mice." *Sleep* 38, no. 1: 31-40. https://doi.org/10.5665/sleep.4320.

Karl, J. Philip, Adrienne M. Hatch, Steven M. Arcidiacono, Sarah C. Pearce, Ida G. Pantoja-Feliciano, Laurel A. Doherty, and Jason W. Soares. 2018. "Effects of Psychological, Environmental and Physical Stressors on the Gut Microbiota." *Frontiers in Microbiology* 9. https://doi.org/10.3389/fmicb.2018.02013.

Kumamoto, Carol A. 2011. "Inflammation and Gastrointestinal Candida Colonization." *Current Opinion in Microbiology* 14, no. 4: 386-391. https://doi.org/10.1016/j.mib.2011.07.015.

Kvietys, Peter R. 2010. "Postprandial Hyperemia." *The Gastrointestinal Circulation*. US National Library of Medicine. In *The Gastrointestinal Circulation*. San Rafael, CA: Morgan & Claypool Life Sciences. https://www.ncbi.nlm.nih.gov/books/NBK53094/.

Li, Hui, Tian He, Qian Xu, Zhe Li, Yan Liu, Fang Li, Bo-Feng Yang, and Cun-Zhi Liu. 2015. "Acupuncture and Regulation of Gastrointestinal Function." *World Journal of Gastroenterology* 21, no. 27: 8304-8313. https://doi.org/10.3748/wjg.v21.i27.8304.

Lurie, Ido, Yu-Xiao Yang, Kevin Haynes, Ronac Mamtani, and Ben Boursi. 2015. "Antibiotic Exposure and the Risk for Depression, Anxiety, or Psychosis." *The Journal of Clinical Psychiatry* 76, no. 11: 1522-28. https://doi.org/10.4088/jcp.15m09961.

Marinac, Catherine R., Sandahl H. Nelson, Caitlin I. Breen, Sheri J. Hartman, Loki Natarajan, John P. Pierce, Shirley W. Flatt, Dorothy D. Sears, and Ruth E. Patterson. 2016. "Prolonged Nightly Fasting and Breast Cancer Prognosis." *JAMA Oncology* 2, no. 8: 1049-1055. https://doi.org/10.1001/jamaoncol.2016.0164.

Maseda, Damian, and Emanuela Ricciotti. 2020. "NSAID-Gut Microbiota Interactions." *Frontiers in Pharmacology* 11: 1-20. https://doi.org/10.3389/fphar.2020.01153.

Nazari, Fatemeh, and Maryam Eghbali. 2012. "Migraine and Its Relationship with Dietary Habits in Women." *Iranian Journal of Nursing and Midwifery Research* 17, no. 2 Suppl 1: S65-71. https://www.ncbi.nlm.nih.gov/pmc/articles/PMC3696968/.

Shang, Hai-Xia, An-Qi Wang, Chun-Hui Bao, Huan-Gan Wu, Wei-Feng Chen, Lu-Yi Wu, Rong Ji, Ji-Meng Zhao, and Yin Shi. 2015. "Moxibustion Combined with Acupuncture Increases Tight Junction Protein Expression in Crohn's Disease Patients." *World Journal of Gastroenterology* 21, no. 16: 4986-4996. https://www.ncbi.nlm.nih.gov/pmc/articles/PMC4408472/.

Tsuchiya, Masahiro, Jun Aida, Yoshihiro Hagiwara, Yumi Sugawara, Yasutake Tomata, Mari Sato, Takashi Watanabe, Hiroaki Tomita, Eiji Nemoto, Makoto Watanabe, Ken Osaka, and Ichiro Tsuji. 2015. "Periodontal Disease Is Associated with Insomnia among Victims of the Great East Japan Earthquake: A Panel

Study Initiated Three Months after the Disaster." *The Tohoku Journal of Experimental Medicine* 237, no. 2: 83-90. https://doi.org/10.1620/tjem.237.83.

Wei, Min, Sebastian Brandhorst, Mahshid Shelehchi, Hamed Mirzaei, Chia Wei Cheng, Julia Budniak, Susan Groshen, Wendy J Mack, Esra Guen, Stefano Di Biase, Pinchas Cohen, Todd E. Morgan, Tanya Dorff, Kurt Hong, Andreas Michalsen, Alessandro Laviano, and Valter D. Longo. 2017. "Fasting-Mimicking Diet and Markers/Risk Factors for Aging, Diabetes, Cancer, and Cardiovascular Disease." *Science Translational Medicine* 9, no. 377: 1-13. https://doi.org/10.1126/scitranslmed.aai8700.

Wiley, T. S. 2000. *Lights Out: Sleep, Sugar, and Survival.* New York: Atria Paperback.

Zuhl, Micah, Karol Dokladny, Christine Mermier, Suzanne Schneider, Roy Salgado, and Pope Moseley. 2015. "The Effects of Acute Oral Glutamine Supplementation on Exercise-Induced Gastrointestinal Permeability and Heat Shock Protein Expression in Peripheral Blood Mononuclear Cells." *Cell Stress and Chaperones* 20, no. 1: 85-93. https://doi.org/10.1007/s12192-014-0528-1.

Chapter 10

Caufriez, Anne, Rachel Leproult, Mireille L'Hermite-Balériaux, Myriam Kerkhofs, and Georges Copinschi. 2011. "Progesterone Prevents Sleep Disturbances and Modulates GH, TSH, and Melatonin Secretion in Postmenopausal Women." *The Journal of Clinical Endocrinology & Metabolism* 96, no. 4: E614-E623. https://doi.org/10.1210/jc.2010-2558.

Endocrine Society. 2018. "Endocrine-Disrupting Chemicals." *Position Statements* (blog). May 1, 2018. https://www.endocrine.org/advocacy/position-statements/endocrine-disrupting-chemicals.

Mulligan, T., M. F. Frick, Q. C. Zuraw, A. Stemhagen, and C. McWhirter. 2006. "Prevalence of Hypogonadism in Males Aged at Least 45 Years: The HIM Study." *International Journal of Clinical Practice* 60, no. 7: 762-769. https://doi.org/10.1111/j.1742-1241.2006.00992.x.

University of Missouri-Columbia. 2011 "Eat A Protein-Rich Breakfast to Reduce Food Cravings, Prevent Overeating Later, Researcher Finds." *Science News* (blog), *ScienceDaily.* May 19, 2011. https://www.sciencedaily.com/releases/2011/05/110519113024.htm.

Watson, Christopher J., Helen A. Baghdoyan, and Ralph Lydic. 2010. "Neuropharmacology of Sleep and Wakefulness." *Sleep Medicine Clinics* 5, no. 4: 513-528. https://www.ncbi.nlm.nih.gov/pmc/articles/PMC3026477/.

Chapter 11

American Thoracic Society. 2017. "Air Pollution May Disrupt Sleep." *Press Releases from the ATS International Conference.* May 21, 2017. https://www.thoracic.org/about/newsroom/press-releases/conference/billings-and-air-pollution-and-sleep.php.

Aristakesian, E. A., L. I. Kiiashchenko, and G. A. Oganesian. 1996. "[The Effect of Cadmium on the Wakefulness-Sleep Cycle in Rats in Early Postnatal Ontogeny]." *Zhurnal Evoliutsionnoi Biokhimii I Fiziologii* 32, no. 4: 402-408. https://pubmed.ncbi.nlm.nih.gov/9054174/.

Benbrook, Charles M. 2019. "How Did the US EPA and IARC Reach Diametrically Opposed Conclusions on The Genotoxicity of Glyphosate-Based Herbicides?" *Environ Sci Eur* 31, no. 2: 1-16. https://doi.org/10.1186/s12302-018-0184-7.

Beydoun, Hind A. May A. Beydoun, Hueiwang Anna Jeng, Alan B. Zonderman, and Shaker M. Eid. 2016. "Bisphenol-A and Sleep Adequacy among Adults in the National Health and Nutrition Examination Surveys." *Sleep* 39, no. 2: 467-476. https://doi.org/10.5665/sleep.5466.

Billings, Martha E., Diane Gold, Adam Szpiro, Carrie P. Aaron, Neal Jorgensen, Amanda Gassett, Peter J. Leary, Joel D. Kaufman, and Susan R. Redline. 2018. "The Association of Ambient Air Pollution with Sleep Apnea: The Multi-Ethnic Study of Atherosclerosis." *Annals of the American Thoracic Society* 16, no. 3: 1-8. https://doi.org/10.1513/annalsats.201804-2480c.

Braestrup, Claus, and Mogens Nielsen. 2003. "Strychnine as a Potent Inhibitor of the Brain GABA/Benzodiazepine Receptor Complex." *Brain Research Bulletin* 5, no. 2: 681-684. https://doi.org/10.1016/0361-9230(80)90112-4.

Cattani, Daiane, Vera Lúcia De Liz Oliveira Cavalli, Carla Elise Heinz Rieg, Juliana Tonietto Domingues, Tharine Dal-Cim, Carla Inês Tasca, Fátima Regina Mena Barreto Silva, and Ariane Zamoner. 2014. "Mechanisms Underlying the Neurotoxicity Induced by Glyphosate-Based Herbicide in Immature Rat Hippocampus: Involvement of Glutamate Excitotoxicity." *Toxicology* 320: 34-45. https://doi.org/10.1016/j.tox.2014.03.001.

Chappell, Bill. 2020. "Bayer to Pay More Than $10 Billion to Resolve Cancer Lawsuits Over Weedkiller Roundup." *Environment* (blog), NPR. June 24, 2022. https://www.npr.org/2020/06/24/882949098/bayer-to-pay-more-than-10-billion-to-resolve-roundup-cancer-lawsuits.

Department of Environmental Protection. 2023. "VOCs: Paints, Cleaners and Other Solvents." *Indoor Air* (blog). https://www.montgomerycountymd.gov/green/air/vocs.html.

Edling, C., A. Lindberg, and J. Ulfberg. 1993. "Occupational Exposure to Organic Solvents as a Cause of Sleep Apnoea." *British*

Journal of Industrial Medicine 50, no. 3: 276-279. https://doi.org/10.1136/oem.50.3.276.

Environmental Protection Agency. 2023a. "Chemical and Products Database (CPDat)." EPA. *Environmental Protection Agency* (blog). March 6, 2023. https://www.epa.gov/chemical-research/chemical-and-products-database-cpdat.

Environmental Protection Agency. 2023b. "Indoor Air Quality." *Report on the Environment* (blog). July 14, 2023. https://www.epa.gov/report-environment/indoor-air-quality.

Environmental Working Group. 2023a. *EWG Skin Deep® Cosmetics Database.* Washington DC: EWG. https://www.ewg.org/skindeep/.

Environmental Working Group. 2023b. "Dirty Dozen: EWG's 2023 Shopper's Guide to Pesticides in Produce". *EWG's 2023 Shopper's Guide to Pesticides in Produce | Dirty Dozen.* https://www.ewg.org/foodnews/dirty-dozen.php.

Foley, Logan. 2023. "Best Organic Mattresses of 2021." *Best Mattress 2023* (blog), *Sleep Foundation.* July 17, 2023. https://www.sleepfoundation.org/best-mattress/best-organic-mattresses.

Geller, Samara. 2022. "Skip the Most Toxic Fabric Softeners." *News Environmental Working Group* (blog). August 16, 2022. https://www.ewg.org/news-insights/news/2022/08/skip-most-toxic-fabric-softeners.

Institute of Medicine of the National Academies. 2014. *Identifying and Reducing Environmental Health Risks of Chemicals in Our Society: Workshop Summary.* Washington DC: The National Academies Press.

Kerr, Kathleen, Gayle Morse, Donald Graves, Fei Zuo, Alain Lipowicz, and David O Carpenter. 2019. "A Detoxification Intervention for Gulf War Illness: A Pilot Randomized Controlled Trial." *International Journal of Environmental Research and Public Health* 16, no. 21: 4143. https://doi.org/10.3390/ijerph16214143.

Li, Jiangping, Yanxing Hao, Danian Tian, Shulan He, Xian Sun, and Huifang Yang. 2019. "Relationship between Cumulative Exposure to Pesticides and Sleep Disorders among Greenhouse Vegetable Farmers." *BMC Public Health* 19, no. 1: 1-11. https://doi.org/10.1186/s12889-019-6712-6.

London, Leslie, Cheryl Beseler, Maryse F. Bouchard, David C. Bellinger, Claudio Colosio, Philippe Grandjean, Raul Harari, Tahira Kootbodien, Hans Kromhout, Francesca Little, Tim Meijster, Angelo Moretto, Diane S. Rohlman, and Lorann Stallones. 2012. "Neurobehavioral and Neurodevelopmental Effects of Pesticide Exposures." *NeuroToxicology* 33, no. 4: 887-896. https://doi.org/10.1016/j.neuro.2012.01.004.

Malin, Ashley J., Sonali Bose, Stefanie A. Busgang, Chris Gennings, Michael Thorpy, Robert O. Wright, Rosalind J. Wright, and Manish Arora. 2019. "Fluoride Exposure and Sleep Patterns among Older Adolescents in the United States: A Cross-Sectional Study of NHANES 2015-2016." *Environmental Health: A Global Access Science Source* 18, no. 1: 106. https://doi.org/10.1186/s12940-019-0546-7.

Malkan, Stacy. 2023. "Glyphosate Fact Sheet: Cancer and Other Health Concerns." *Pesticides* (blog). *US Right to Know*. March 17, 2023. https://usrtk.org/pesticides/glyphosate-health-concerns/.

Mayo Clinic Staff. 2022. "Lead Poisoning." *Mayo Foundation for Medical Education and Research* (blog), Mayo Clinic. Jan 21, 2022. https://www.mayoclinic.org/diseases-conditions/lead-poisoning/symptoms-causes/syc-20354717.

McManus, Katherine D. 2019. "Should I Be Eating More Fiber?" *Harvard Health Blog* (blog), Harvard Health Publishing. February 27, 2019. https://www.health.harvard.edu/blog/should-i-be-eating-more-fiber-2019022115927.

Minnesota Department of Health. 2022. "Volatile Organic Compounds (VOCs) in Your Home." *Indoor Air* (blog). November 20, 2022. https://www.health.state.mn.us/communities/environment/air/toxins/voc.htm.

Myers, John Peterson, Michael N. Antoniou, Bruce Blumberg, Lynn Carroll, Theo Colborn, Lorne G. Everett, Michael Hansen, Philip J. Landrigan, Bruce P. Lanphear, Robin Mesnage, Laura N. Vandenberg, Frederick S. vom Saal, Wade V. Welshons and Charles M. Benbrook. 2016. "Concerns over Use of Glyphosate-Based Herbicides and Risks Associated with Exposures: A Consensus Statement." *Environmental Health* 15, no. 1: 1-13. https://doi.org/10.1186/s12940-016-0117-0.

New York Daily News. 2013. "Exercise Prevents Painful Kidney Stones in Women over 50, Large Study Finds." *Daily Health* (blog). May 3, 2013. https://www.nydailynews.com/life-style/health/exercise-prevents-painful-kidney-stones-women-article-1.1334156.

Oz, Kira, Bareket Merav, Sabach Sara, and Dubowski Yael. 2019. "Volatile Organic Compound Emissions from Polyurethane Mattresses under Variable Environmental Conditions." *Environmental Science & Technology* 53, no. 15: 9171-9180. https://doi.org/10.1021/acs.est.9b01557.

Pizzorno, Joseph. 2015. "The Kidney Dysfunction Epidemic, Part 1: Causes." *Integrative Medicine* 14, no. 6: 8-13. https://www.ncbi.nlm.nih.gov/pmc/articles/PMC4718206/.

Postuma, R. B., J. Y. Montplaisir, A. Pelletier, Y. Dauvilliers, W. Oertel, A. Iranzo, L. Ferini-Strambi, I. Arnulf, B. Hogl, R. Manni, T. Miyamoto, G. Mayer, K. Stiasny-Kolster, M. Puligheddu, Y. Ju, P. Jennum, K. Sonka, J. Santamaria, M. L. Fantini, M. Zucconi, S. Leu-Semenescu, B. Frauscher, M. Terzaghi, M. Miyamoto, M. M. Unger, V. Cochen De Cock, and C. Wolfson. 2012. "Environmental Risk Factors for REM Sleep Behavior Disorder: A Multicenter Case-Control Study." *Neurology* 79, no. 5: 428-434. https://doi.org/10.1212/wnl.0b013e31825dd383.

Rossini, Sueli Regina G., Rubens Reimão, Beatriz H. Lefèvre, and Marcília A. Medrado-Faria. 2000. "Chronic Insomnia in Workers Poisoned by Inorganic Mercury: Psychological and Adaptive Aspects." *Associação Arquivos de Neuro-Psiquiatria* 58, no. 1: 32-28. https://doi.org/10.1590/S0004-282X2000000100005.

Samsel, Anthony, and Stephanie Seneff. 2013. "Glyphosate, Pathways to Modern Diseases II: Celiac Sprue and Gluten Intolerance." *Interdisciplinary Toxicology* 6, no. 4: 159-84. https://doi.org/10.2478/intox-2013-0026.

Sears, Margaret E., Kerr J. Kathleen, and Bray I. Riina. 2012. "Arsenic, Cadmium, Lead, and Mercury in Sweat: A Systematic Review." *Journal of Environmental and Public Health* 2012: 1-10. https://doi.org/10.1155/2012/184745.

Shiue, Ivy. 2016. "Urinary Arsenic, Pesticides, Heavy Metals, Phthalates, Polyaromatic Hydrocarbons, and Polyfluoroalkyl Compounds Are Associated with Sleep Troubles in Adults: USA NHANES, 2005-2006." *Environmental Science and Pollution Research* 24, no. 3: 3108-3116. https://doi.org/10.1007/s11356-016-8054-6.

Shiue, Ivy. 2017. "Urinary Arsenic, Pesticides, Heavy Metals, Phthalates, Polyaromatic Hydrocarbons, And Polyfluoroalkyl Compounds Are Associated with Sleep Troubles in Adults: USA NHANES, 2005-2006." *Environ Sci Pollut Res* 24: 3108-3116. https://doi.org/10.1007/s11356-016-8054-6.

Unde, Maitreyee P, Raju Umaji Patil, and Persis P Dastoor. 2018. "The Untold Story of Fluoridation: Revisiting the Changing Perspectives." *Indian Journal of Occupational and Environmental Medicine* 22, no. 3: 121-127. https://www.ncbi.nlm.nih.gov/pmc/articles/PMC6309358/.

Chapter 12

Babatunde, Shola Kola, Abayomi Fadeyi, Ajibola Ahmed Akanbi II, Charles Nwabuisi, and Yemi Jimoh Abdulraheem. 2013. "Cyclosporiasis and Other Intestinal Parasitoses in Association with Diarrhoea in Ilorin, Nigeria." *African Journal of Microbiology Research* 7, no. 21: 2613-2617. https://doi.org/10.5897/ajmr2013.5583.

Buhner, Stephen Harrod. 2015. *Healing Lyme*. New York, NY: Raven Press.

Buhner, Stephen Harrod. 2013. *Healing Lyme Disease Coinfections: Complementary and Holistic Treatments for Bartonella and Mycoplasma*. Rochester, VT: Healing Arts Press.

El-Zawawy, Hanaa Tarek and Huda Fahmy Farag. 2020. "Improving Hashimoto's Thyroiditis by Eradicating *Blastocystis hominis*: Relation to IL-17." *Therapeutic Advances in Endocrinology and Metabolism* 11. https://doi.org/10.1177/2042018820907013.

National Institutes of Health. 2018. "Epstein-Barr Virus Protein Can 'Switch on' Risk Genes for Autoimmune Diseases." *News Releases* (blog), US Department of Health and Human Services. April 16, 2018. https://www.nih.gov/news-events/news-releases/epstein-barr-virus-protein-can-switch-risk-genes-autoimmune-diseases.

Nathan, Neil. 2018. *Toxic: Heal Your Body from Mold Toxicity, Lyme Disease, Multiple Chemical Sensitivities, and Chronic Environmental Illness*. Las Vegas, NV: Victory Belt Publishing.

Naviaux, Robert K. 2014. "Metabolic Features of the Cell Danger Response." *Mitochondrion* 16: 7-17. https://doi.org/10.1016/j.mito.2013.08.006.

Sanchez, Albert, J. L. Reeser, H. S. Lau, P. Y. Yahiku, R. E. Willard, P. J. McMillan, S. Y. Cho, A. R. Magie, and U. D. Register. 1973. "Role of Sugars in Human Neutrophilic Phagocytosis."

The American Journal of Clinical Nutrition, 26, no. 11: 1180-1184. https://doi.org/10.1093/ajcn/26.11.1180.
Shoemaker, Ritchie C. 2010. *Surviving Mold: Life in the Era of Dangerous Buildings*. Baltimore, MD: Otter Bay Books, LLC.
Surviving Mold. n.d. "Ritchie Shoemaker, M. D." *About Dr. Ritchie Shoemaker, M.D.* (blog). https://www.survivingmold.com/about/ritchie-shoemaker-m-d.
Valtonen, Ville. 2017. "Clinical Diagnosis of the Dampness and Mold Hypersensitivity Syndrome: Review of the Literature and Suggested Diagnostic Criteria." *Frontiers in Immunology* 8. https://doi.org/10.3389/fimmu.2017.00951.
Vezir, Sedat, Filiz Kaya, Emine Vezir, Nermin Karaosmanoğlu, and Ali Kudret Adiloğlu. 2019. "Evaluation of Intestinal Parasites in Patients with Chronic Spontaneous Urticaria in a Territory Hospital in Turkey." *The Journal of Infection in Developing Countries* 13, no. 10: 927-932. https://doi.org/10.3855/jidc.11552.
Wedi, Bettina, Ulrike Raap, Dorothea Wieczorek, and Alexander Kapp. 2009. "Urticaria and Infections." *Allergy, Asthma & Clinical Immunology* 5, no. 10: 1-12. https://doi.org/10.1186/1710-1492-5-10.

Chapter 14

Institute of Medicine (US) Committee on Military Nutrition Research. 1970. *Caffeine for the Sustainment of Mental Task Performance.* Washington DC: National Academy Press.
University of Missouri-Columbia. 2011. "Eat A Protein-Rich Breakfast to Reduce Food Cravings, Prevent Overeating Later, Researcher Finds." *Science News* (blog), *ScienceDaily.* May 19, 2011. https://www.sciencedaily.com/releases/2011/05/110519113024.htm.

Chapter 15

American College of Cardiology. 2019. "A Nap A Day Keeps High Blood Pressure at Bay: Catching Some Midday Shut-Eye Linked to Similar Drops in Blood Pressure Seen with Other Lifestyle Changes, Some Medications." *Science News* (blog), *ScienceDaily.* March 7, 2019. www.sciencedaily.com/releases/2019/03/190307081029.htm.

Pacheco, Danielle, and Heather Wright. 2023. "The Best Temperature for Sleep: Advice & Tips." *Sleep Foundation* (blog). July 12, 2023. https://www.sleepfoundation.org/bedroom-environment/best-temperature-for-sleep.

Printed in Great Britain
by Amazon